# FACE FOOD

DISCOVER HOW FACE LIFTING FOOD CAN
BOOST YOUR COLLAGEN AND TAKE YEARS
OFF YOUR FACE NATURALLY

## GREGORY LANDSMAN

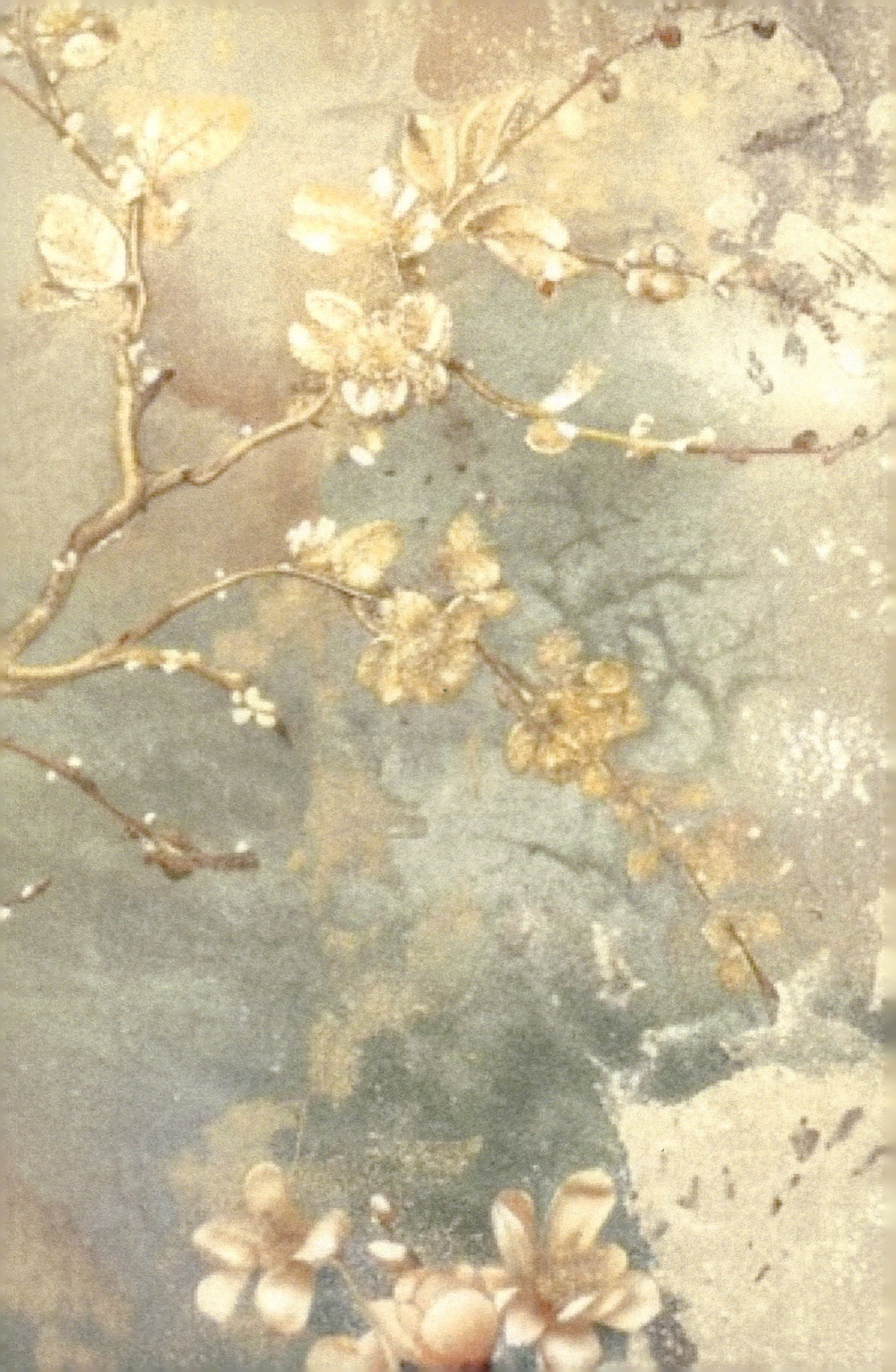

Copyright 2010 © Gregory Landsman Reprinted 2018, 2020, 2022, 2024

*Published in the United States* by Hill of Content Publishing

*Published in the United Kingdom* by Hill of Content Publishing

*Published in Australia* by Hill of Content Publishing

*Published in India* by Hill of Content Publishing

hillofcontentpublishing.com

PO Box 24 East Melbourne 8002 Victoria Australia

All rights reserved. No part of this publication may be reproduced, stored in a retrieval system or transmitted in any form by any means without the prior permission of the copyright owner. Enquiries should be made to the publisher. Every effort has been made to ensure that this book is free from error or omissions. However, the Publisher, the Author, the Editor or their respective employees or agents, shall not accept responsibility for injury, loss or damage occasioned to any person acting or refraining from action as a result of material in this book whether or not such injury, loss or damage is in any way due to any negligent act or omission, breach of duty or default on the part of the Publisher, the Author, the Editor, or their respective employees or agents. The Author, the Publisher, the Editor and their respective employees or agents do not accept any responsibility for the actions of any person - actions which are related in any way to information contained in this book.

Landsman, Gregory

Face Food: Discover how Face Lifting Food can boost your collagen and take years off your face naturally.

ISBN: 978-0-6482892-2-7

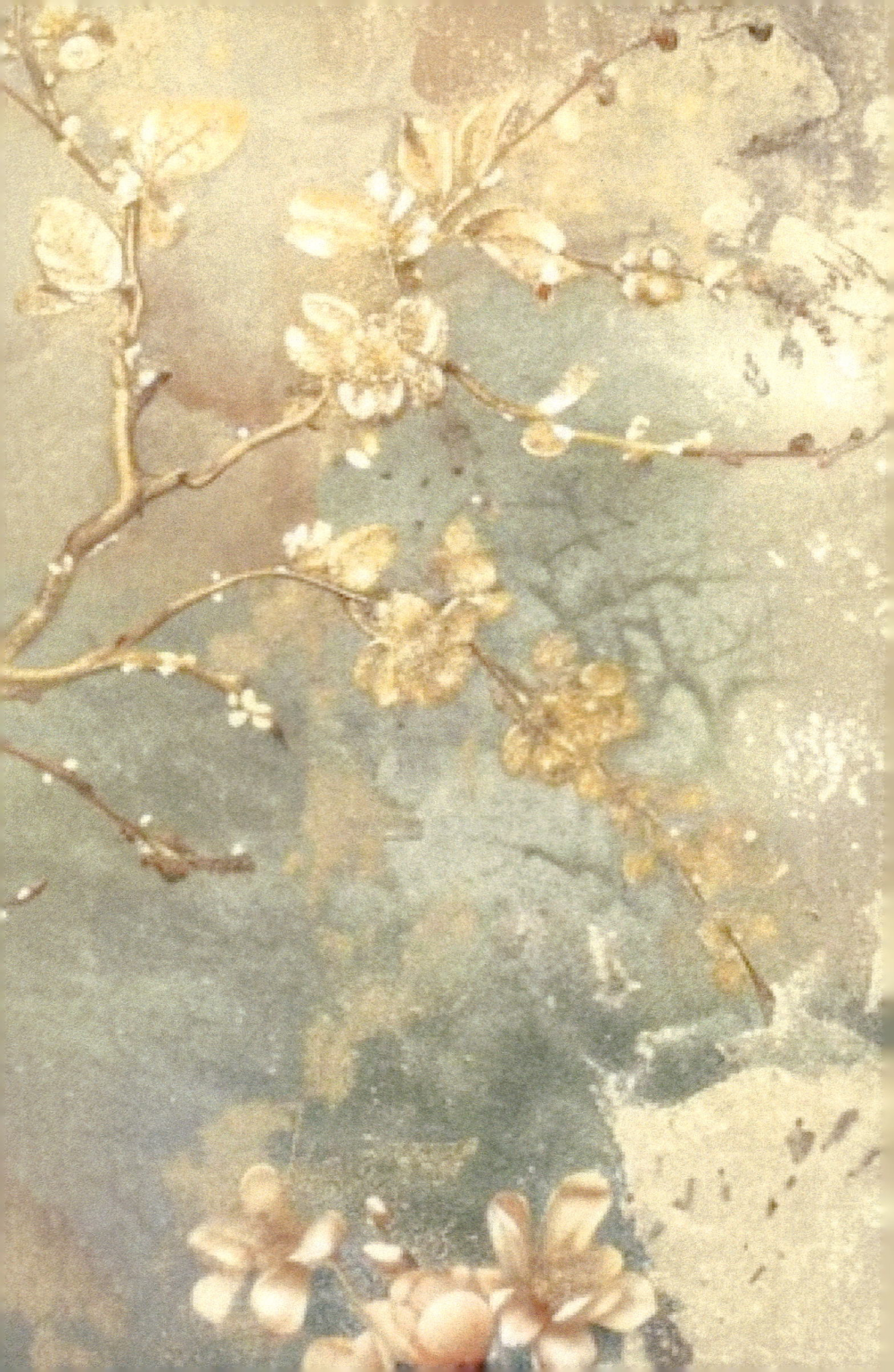

# FROM THE AUTHOR

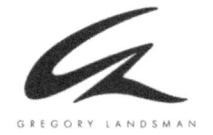

GREGORY LANDSMAN

*While our skin undergoes many changes in our lifetime, food is a powerful transformational element that we can use to counteract skin stress and achieve firmer, healthier, younger looking skin at any age.*

What I am going to show you in this book is that simple, tasty foods have the ability to flush your face with vitality, improve and change the quality and texture of your skin, reduce wrinkles and fine lines, increase firmness and combat premature aging. How? With the right foods we can counteract skin stress, supporting the body's natural ability to eliminate and neutralise toxins, which ensures optimal skin functioning and collagen production.

While genetic factors play a major role in the way we age, so does the food that we eat. In fact our diet is one of the great age-defying secrets to retaining or regaining healthy, vital looking skin. It's all based on the basic principal that we need to detox our system to support the skin to build and protect its collagen. This is the foundation of healthy, youthful looking skin; as when we increase collagen, skin regains its elasticity.

Dealing with faces every day as I have for many years, it is easy to see when skin has been deprived of nutrients. So whenever I recommend a skin solution I keep in mind that one of the most effective ways to protect and preserve our skin at any age involves eating the right skin renewing foods.

Many of the natural foods we eat hold vitamins and minerals that are essential to give your skin radiance, while supporting, hydrating and maintaining the health of the skin. They are also the key to helping the body counteract skin stress so it can function optimally - eliminating toxins and building collagen.

You may ask why building collagen is so important? Simply because collagen is the protein in connective tissue that keeps the skin elastic. However, the fibres in these tissues can become weak and damaged through free radicals, which impact our skin both inside and out as a result of different lifestyle elements such as stress, toxins, fast food, sugar, sun damage, smoking, alcohol and the list goes on!

However collagen cannot be absorbed from a beauty cream as the molecules are too large to penetrate the skin's cells. This means the most effective solution is either topically applying (see Face Value) or eating foods full of skin regenerating vitamins and minerals that naturally renew, stimulate and protect collagen.

For example Vitamin C is a powerful antioxidant that protects and stabilises collagen; Vitamin K supports skin healing; Vitamin E regenerates and smoothes skin; Vitamin

A builds collagen fibres and exfoliates skin; and Copper firms the skin and enhances its elasticity.

The quick and easy recipes in this book are power packed with skin building ingredients (antioxidants, vitamins and essential minerals) to counteract skin stress, while naturally building and stimulating your body's collagen and increasing the health, thickness and firmness of the skin.

Alternatively, you can create your own recipes using the Face Lifting Food list at the back of the book. Once you are familiar with the skin boosting foods that support your skin, you will be able to incorporate them into some of your favourite dishes.

I developed the recipes and detox cleanse in Face Food, as my own eating plan to support overall health and wellbeing. Please keep in mind that this is not a program for specific ailments. If you do have health concerns please consult your doctor before commencing the 5-Day Skin Detox Cleanse.

While food enhances our experience of life, since ancient times it has been a powerful source of cleansing and healing. Cooking is not only a wonderful reminder that sharing food with those we love nurtures their health and skin from the inside out, but that the true essence of our beauty is in sharing the spirit of our humanity in all that we do.

My personal wellbeing philosophy is...

**B alance** in our life unfolds from the inside out.

**E nthusiasm** lies within the way we think and feel about ourselves.

**A cceptance** is the path to making peace with ourselves and others.

**U nderstanding** ourselves gives us clarity and wisdom to know what we want, and importantly, what we don't.

**T rust** attunes our heart and mind so we can nurture spontaneity and adventure in our lives, and see that...

**Y ou** have what it takes to create the life and love you know you deserve and to never settle for anything less.

So while our skin is the largest organ in the body and we need to look after it, it is important to remain true to our beauty by never forgetting that laughter and humour play a major role in experiencing and feeling it.

*After all the beauty we feel is the beauty we live.*

GREGORY LANDSMAN

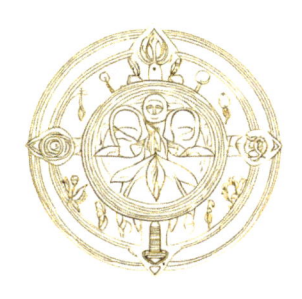

*Our skin feels like it is always shouting, 'Look at me!' But what it is really showing us is the way we eat, the amount of water we are drinking, the quality of our daily breathing, how much sleep we have had and the stress we are living with.*

*If your face is a map of your life, your skin is a daily reminder of your stress levels and your lifestyle staring back at you.*

— GREGORY LANDSMAN

## CONTENTS

| | |
|---|---|
| FROM THE AUTHOR | 1 |
| SKIN FIRMING BOOSTERS | 13 |
| 8 Super Skin Firming Vitamins That Can Nourish, Revitalise And Protect Your Skin | 14 |
| 7 Powerful Skin Firming Minerals To Tighten, Brighten And Change The Quality Of Your Skin | 20 |
| 9 Essential Skin Firming Nutrients To Perk And Plump Skin | 26 |
| Fast Effective Skin Firming Reminders | 30 |
| 5-DAY SKIN DETOX CLEANSE | 33 |
| FACE LIFTING FOOD BREAKFAST OPTIONS | 43 |
| Collagen Building Smoothie | 44 |
| Skin Rejuvenating Tossed Fruit | 45 |
| Antioxidant Hot Porridge | 47 |
| Skin Boosting Muesli | 48 |
| Anti-inflammatory Egg Omelette | 50 |
| Radiant Skin Watermelon Refresher | 52 |
| Skin Moisturising Avocado on Wholegrain Toast | 53 |
| Skin Strengthening Berry & Yogurt Mix | 55 |
| FACE LIFTING FOOD LUNCH OPTIONS | 57 |
| Skin Plumping Sardine Bruschetta | 58 |
| Vitamin E Loaded Salad Dressing | 60 |
| Calcium Rich Veggie Frittata | 62 |
| Potassium Filled Tuna Potatoes | 64 |
| Vitamin A Skin Renewing Smoked Trout Salad | 66 |
| A & C Skin Building Pea Soup | 68 |
| Collagen Corn And Pepper Soup | 70 |
| 'C' Bean Salad | 72 |

| | |
|---|---|
| Potassium Packed Spanish Salad | 74 |
| Skin Building Spiced Cauliflower | 76 |
| Nurturing Antioxidant Avocado Citrus Salad | 78 |
| FACE LIFTING FOOD DINNER OPTIONS | 81 |
| Skin Illuminating Mackerel With Salad | 82 |
| Collagen Building Poached Fish (Or Chicken) | 84 |
| Skin Protecting Chicken With Vegetables | 86 |
| Super Skin Antioxidant Salmon With Coconut | 88 |
| Antioxidant Salmon (Or Chicken) With Teriyaki Sauce | 90 |
| Wrinkle Prevention Fish (Or Chicken) Kebabs | 92 |
| FACE LIFTING FOOD SNACK OPTIONS | 95 |
| Points To Remember For Tighter, Brighter, Healthier Skin | 96 |
| FACE LIFTING FOOD LIST | 98 |
| THE BALANCE OF BEAUTY PHILOSOPHY | 107 |
| THE FOUR PILLARS OF SKIN HEALTH TO DE-STRESS & AGE LESS | |
| About Gregory Landsman | 118 |
| Connect with Gregory Landsman | 119 |

# THE TRUTH ABOUT HOW SKIN AGES

**If you are serious about looking younger, reducing fine lines and wrinkles, improving skin hydration, and getting a natural glow back then you need to understand how skin stress ages the skin.**

## SKIN STRESS HAPPENS TO MOST PEOPLE EVERY DAY REGARDLESS OF THEIR SKINCARE ROUTINE

Every day as part of daily life we are exposed to toxins that impact the skin. Skin stress is brought on by the toxins we consume and are exposed to as a result of our lifestyle choices, that dry the skin and cause it to age prematurely. This includes what we eat, how we breathe, the skincare we use, the cosmetics we apply every day, the sugar we consume, the amount of alcohol we drink, whether we smoke, our level of sun exposure; and the stress we carry day-to-day.

When we are feeling stressed, the adrenal glands release the stress hormone known as cortisol. When this happens, sugar levels in the blood naturally increase, and the increased blood sugar promotes 'glycation' in our skin and damages our collagen and elastin - the skin's building blocks that give it structure and keep it firm and elastic. Damaged collagen equals an increase in skin dryness, wrinkles and premature aging.

**When cortisol is raging you are aging prematurely!** Cortisol decreases our skin's natural production of hyaluronic acid, which acts as a natural moisturiser for our skin. This allows even more hydration to be lost; and when skin is dehydrated, the enzymes in our skin that work to repair the damage don't work as well.

## THE SKIN STRESS CYCLE WEAKENS AND AGES THE SKIN

This daily dose of skin stress in so many forms creates a skin stress cycle that weakens skin, compromises skin hydration, creates free radicals and destroys collagen. This results in a sallow dull, dry, complexion, increases fine lines and wrinkles, and ages the skin prematurely.

## WE NEED MORE THAN SKINCARE PRODUCTS TO BREAK THE SKIN STRESS CYCLE

It's not enough to just have a good skincare routine and stay out of the sun. Skincare products and creams do not always have the skin building nutrients to counteract skin stress created by daily living, which is why you may be paying good money and doing everything right, but still not getting the results you'd like.

## THE SOLUTION TO ENJOYING GLOWING SKIN AT EVERY AGE IS BREAKING THE SKIN STRESS CYCLE

If we want to look as good as we can for as long as we can, we need to break the cycle and counteract daily skin stress, so we can naturally age less! To do this we need to get our skin health functioning at optimal levels, fortifying the body's defence system and simultaneously supporting collagen production.

There are a myriad of things that create skin stress and age the skin prematurely. However, once you understand what creates skin stress, good skincare must incorporate proactive skin stress reduction.

While we all want to age gracefully, there is no harm in giving grace a helping hand. So regardless of how old you are, whether you have just noticed your first line, or they have been etched firmly into your skin for decades, when the skin is stressed we will visibly see signs of premature aging that will show as a loss of skin tone, a dull complexion, skin dryness or fine lines and wrinkles.

My approach is simple, effective and natural, and now in my sixties I have practiced it daily for decades. I will show you how to strengthen your skin, stimulate your skin fitness and elevate your overall wellbeing, so you can feel good and look good.

In Face Food I show you how to:

- Stimulate and protect collagen
- Tighten skin and improve elasticity

- Reduce fine lines and wrinkles
- Protect skin with natural antioxidants
- Increase the thickness and suppleness of skin
- Restore skin radiance

Breaking the skin stress cycle will put back the purity and goodness into your skin that day to day living takes out and show you how to maintain healthy glowing, radiant skin at every age.

*The key to maintaining skin health over a lifetime is to make small changes that reduce skin stress and deliver big skin results when practised regularly.*

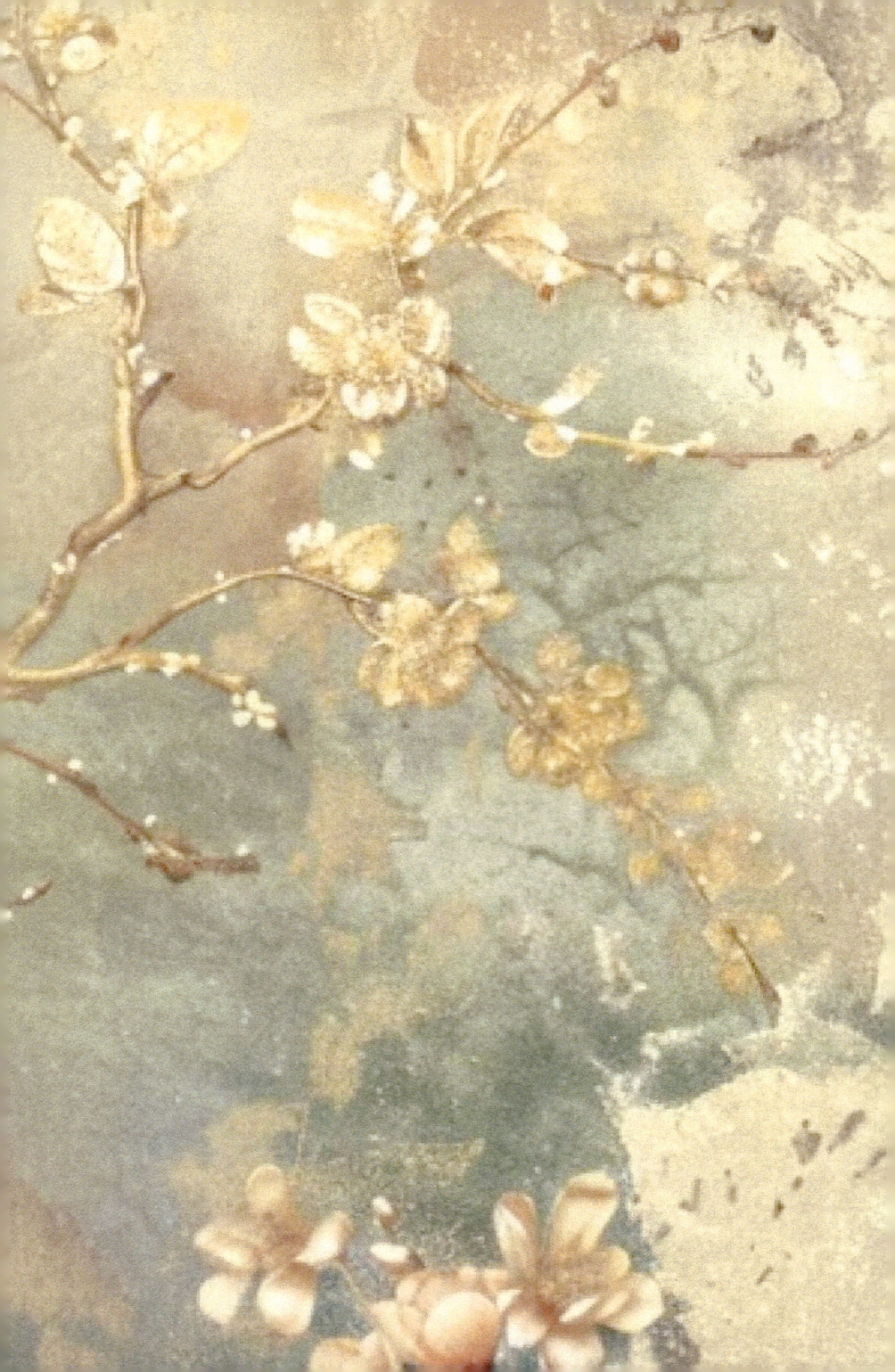

# SKIN FIRMING BOOSTERS

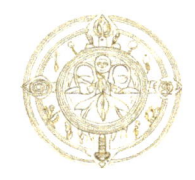

**Some of the most powerful skin renewing ingredients found in the most exclusive anti-aging creams such as Coenzyme Q10, Vitamins C, A and E, can all be found in the foods that we eat.**

While applying vitamins topically to your skin can have a visible impact, consuming the right nutrients can bring about positive lasting changes to your skin. When it comes to the beauty of our skin it is important to monitor and become conscious of the foods we eat.

While free radicals break down healthy skin tissue, consuming the right foods can counter act that. You will be amazed at how making the right food choices can overhaul the look and feel of your skin. In the following pages you will find some of the key skin boosting ingredients to include in your diet regularly.

# 8 SUPER SKIN FIRMING VITAMINS THAT CAN NOURISH, REVITALISE AND PROTECT YOUR SKIN

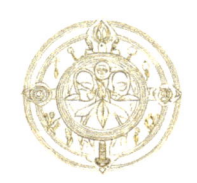

VITAMIN A

Vitamin A is a power vitamin for skin with strong anti-aging benefits. It is an antioxidant that helps the skin stay strong, smooth and firm while increasing elasticity.

If Vitamin A levels are low a variety of skin issues can occur including dryness and flaking.

**Foods with Vitamin A include:**

- Baked sweet potatoes, peeled pumpkin
- Beef liver
- Spinach
- Cantaloupe
- Peas and carrots

## VITAMIN C

**Vitamin C** is key to collagen production and protection, but as it cannot be stored in the body it needs to be topped up and included regularly in your diet.

Vitamin C helps to counteract the skin's exposure to sun and fights free radicals that induce wrinkles by destroying collagen and elastin fibres that support the structure of the skin.

**Ensure your diet is rich in Vitamin C foods such as:**

- Strawberries
- Orange
- Grapefruit
- Lemon
- Cantaloupe
- Tomato
- Cucumber

Foods that carry greater doses of Vitamin C than oranges include:

- Blackcurrants (4x)
- Red peppers (4x)
- Parsley (3x)
- Kiwifruit and Brussels sprouts (1.9x)
- Broccoli (1.8x)

## VITAMIN E

**Vitamin E** is a powerful antioxidant that protects and reduces the damage caused to skin cells from sun exposure.

It is also an anti-inflammatory that helps to soothe and smooth the texture of the skin and reduce wrinkles.

**Foods high in Vitamin E include:**

- Fish
- Wheat germ oil
- Almonds
- Sunflower seeds, dry roasted
- Sunflower oil
- Safflower oil
- Hazelnuts, dry roasted
- Peanut butter
- Peanuts, dry roasted
- Green leafy vegetables like spinach
- Broccoli
- Soybean oil
- Mango

## VITAMIN B

**Vitamin B Complex** has a variety of B vitamins that are great for the skin.

Good sources of group B vitamins include:

- Chicken and turkey
- Red meats
- Fish

- Eggs
- Whole wheat breads
- Rice
- Soy
- Corn

More specifically, **B7** or **Biotin** is one of the most important nutrients that forms skin, nail and hair cells. While the body makes plenty of this B Vitamin, eating Biotin rich foods can give skin a healthy glow. Applying it topically can also improve the texture and overall tone of the skin while hydrating cells.

**Foods high in B7 include:**

- Bananas
- Eggs
- Oatmeal
- Rice

**B3 is another essential B vitamin for skin.**

Known as **Niacin**, **B3** supports skin to retain moisture, helping skin look more youthful and plump. It also has strong anti-inflammatory properties that help soothe irritated and dry skin.

**Niacin rich foods include:**

- All lean red meats
- Fish
- Organ meats (kidney, liver)
- Prawns
- Pork

- Milk (and other dairy products)
- Almonds
- Seeds
- Wheat products
- Beans
- Rice bran
- Green leafy vegetables
- Carrots
- Turnips
- Celery

VITAMIN D

**Vitamin D** is a large contributor to cell metabolism and growth and helps the body absorb important skin building vitamins, phosphorous and magnesium.

**Foods with Vitamin D include:**

- Beef
- Milk
- Cheese
- Cod liver oil
- Eggs
- Liver
- Mackerel
- Salmon
- Sardines
- Tuna

## VITAMIN K

**Vitamin K** is effective in reducing bruising and under eye circles.

**Foods high in Vitamin K include:**

- Parsley
- Avocado
- Nectarine
- Papaya
- Peach
- Pear
- Plum
- Strawberries
- Asparagus
- Bok Choy
- Broccoli
- Brussels sprouts
- Cabbage
- Zucchini
- Green peppers
- Olive oil
- Carrots
- Spinach

# 7 POWERFUL SKIN FIRMING MINERALS TO TIGHTEN, BRIGHTEN AND CHANGE THE QUALITY OF YOUR SKIN

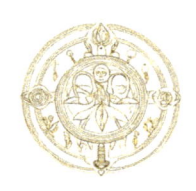

## MAGNESIUM

**Magnesium** promotes circulation and is vital for repairing and maintaining the health of cells. It slows down the aging process, ensuring healthy elasticity is maintained and moisture levels remain normal.

**Good sources of Magnesium include:**

- Brown rice
- Wheat bran
- Almonds
- Avocado
- Banana
- Green vegetables (particularly Spinach)
- Milk
- Yoghurt
- Oatmeal

ZINC

**Zinc** is a skin firming and strengthening mineral (preventing wrinkles) required for collagen production and elastic synthesis.

**Good sources of Zinc include:**

- Seafood
- Turkey
- Oysters
- Poultry
- Mushrooms
- Soy beans
- Lean meat
- Beef liver
- Lima beans
- Chickpeas
- Split peas
- Cashews (raw)
- Pecans (raw)
- Green peas
- Ginger root
- Organic eggs

SELENIUM

**Selenium** helps to prevent tissue damage caused by free radicals and can help protect the skin from sun damage.

**Good sources of Selenium include:**

- Garlic

- Eggs
- Seafood (including cooked oysters)
- Cereal/ wholegrains
- Fish
- Sunflower seeds
- Chilli peppers
- Tuna light, canned oil
- Beef
- Turkey
- Chicken
- Cottage cheese
- Oatmeal
- Rice (white and brown)
- Walnuts
- Brazil nuts

COPPER

**Copper** is an essential skin building mineral which helps to produce elastin fibres that support the underlying skin structure.

**Most fruits contain a small amount of copper and some good sources include:**

- Barley
- Whole wheat breads
- Beans
- Peas
- Lentils
- Black eyed peas
- Soy beans
- Almonds and cashews

- English walnuts
- Pine and Brazil nuts
- Peanuts
- Pistacchio
- Mushrooms
- Potato
- Sweet potato
- Tomato juice
- Prunes
- Turnips
- Beef
- Chicken
- Turkey
- Clams
- Crab meat
- Shrimp
- Pumpkin seeds
- Sunflower seeds

## CALCIUM

**Calcium** is a wonder mineral for the skin that helps stop visible aging. It not only assists in protecting the skin against moisture loss, it is key to maintaining skin thickness (or plumpness), while stimulating production of the skin's own age protective antioxidants.

**Good sources of Calcium include:**

- Broccoli
- Dairy products
- Leafy green vegetables
- Salmon

- Sardines
- Soy milk
- Tofu

## PHOSPHORUS

**Phosphorus** contributes to the repair and maintenance of body cells.

**Good sources of Phosphorus include:**

- Beans
- Peas
- Bran flakes
- Whole wheat bread
- Sunflower seeds
- Broccoli
- Corn
- Potato
- Fish
- Green leafy vegetables
- Milk
- Yoghurt

## POTASSIUM

**Potassium** is essential for the body's growth and maintenance, ensuring a normal water balance between the cells.

**High sources of Potassium include:**

- All poultry

- Fish
- Avocado
- Banana
- Cantaloupe
- Lima beans
- Milk
- Orange
- Kiwifruit
- Potato
- Plums
- Spinach
- Tomato

# 9 ESSENTIAL SKIN FIRMING NUTRIENTS TO PERK AND PLUMP SKIN

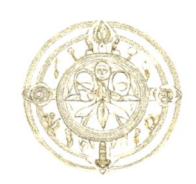

ESSENTIAL FATTY ACIDS

**Essential fatty acids such as Omega 3 and 6** are essential for dewy skin as it helps the production of the skin's natural oil barrier which keeps skin youthful and smoother.

**Omega 3 fatty acid (Linoleic acid)** is an essential fat that plumps skin up and makes it look and feel younger.

- Flaxseed oil (highest content)
- Goji berries
- Walnuts
- Sesame seeds
- Pumpkin Seeds
- Soybean oil
- Salmon
- Mackerel
- Sardines
- Anchovies

- Avocados
- Dark green lettuce
- Brazil nuts
- Sunflower oil
- Sesame oil

**Oleic acid** is skin boosting with strong antioxidant properties along with natural anti-inflammatory properties. It helps the cells absorb essential fatty acids effectively and research has shown that it reduces the appearance of fine lines and wrinkles by penetrating and plumping the skin cell membranes.

Good sources of Oleic acid include:

- Avocado
- Olive Oil
- Nuts
- Olives

## COENZYME Q10

**Coenzyme Q10** is an antioxidant that protects against oxidative damage from free radicals. The body produces its own Coenzyme Q10, however this can be impacted by both age and stress.

**Good sources of Coenzyme Q10 include:**

- Sardines, Tuna and Mackerel
- Cabbage
- Spinach
- Peanuts

DMAE

**DMAE** is a potent antioxidant that fights free radicals and prevents the formation of the brown pigment which becomes the basis for age spots. When eaten regularly it can increase muscle tone and reduce the appearance of sagging.

**DMAE can be found in salmon and anchovies.**

ANTHOCYANINS
**Anthocyanins** are found in all purple foods and help support skin and collagen production.

**Good sources of Anthocyanins include:**

- Beetroot
- Red cabbage
- Red onions

HYALURONIC ACID

**Hyaluronic acid** plumps and smooths skin. As this decreases naturally with age, consuming foods with Hyaluronic acid is important.

**Good sources include most beans (from baked beans, to butter or kidney beans).**

LUTEIN

**Lutein** boosts skin hydration, elasticity and combats wrinkles.

**Foods high in Lutein are:**

- Broccoli
- Peas
- Brussels sprouts
- Sweet corn
- Green beans
- Egg yolk

## CARNOSINE

**Carnosine** is an important skin building protein that slows a process in the skin called cross linking. When this happens fibres grow into the collagen which reduces elasticity. This impacts on the skin snapping back when you do things like smile, laugh or frown.

**Good sources of Carnosine are:**

- Milk
- Eggs
- Poultry

# FAST EFFECTIVE SKIN FIRMING REMINDERS

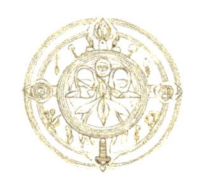

*Your skin is an expression of your health,
vitality and the foods you consume.*

While knowing what foods support our skin is important, we must also take into consideration the foods and behaviours that threaten the health of our skin.

**Avoid Crash Diets** as you lose lean muscle tissue, which causes skin to sag and the face to become drawn. Losing weight gradually allows your skin to shrink gently, so the elastin and collagen fibres can become accustomed to the change.

**To Avoid Inflammation of the Skin** reduce salt and eliminate white flour, rice, pasta and sugar. Also eliminate processed foods as they are loaded with sugar and additives that rob the skin of essential nutrients. Sugar also causes premature aging as it blocks Vitamin C functions, which are essential for collagen and elastin production.

For best results cut out coffee and all dairy products (with the exception of low-fat yoghurt) from your diet.

**Use Sea Salt** (good quality, hand harvested – usually found at health food stores), as it contains potassium, magnesium and calcium, which are all essential skin building nutrients.

## KEEP IN MIND WHEN MAKING THE FACE LIFTING FOOD RECIPES...

**Garlic:** To access the powerful allicin sulphur compound found in garlic it is essential that to chop or crush it and let it sit for ten minutes before using it. Or you can eat it raw for maximum benefits. Allicin can increase the skin's antioxidant levels; support more nutrients to be delivered to the skin through increased blood circulation; and smooth the skin. It is also anti-inflammatory and anti-microbial.

**Greens:** Pouring olive oil over green vegetables helps the body benefit from the nutrients as the vitamins in greens are absorbed more effectively when consumed with fat.

**Tomatoes:** Cooking tomatoes for 30 minutes helps increase the levels of lycopene by more than 50%. Lycopene is a powerful antioxidant which helps the body fight free radicals and supports skin hydration, skin elasticity, firmness and texture. Adding olive oil helps the body to absorb it more effectively.

**Asparagus, Avocado, cabbage, and cauliflower** contain glutathione, known as the master of all antioxidants as it improves moisture levels, skin tone, smoothness and skin elasticity, while reducing fine lines and wrinkles. It can also help counteract hyperpigmentation and sun damage.

**Onions, soybeans, seafood, turkey, nuts:** Contain sulphur, known as the beauty mineral because it boosts collagen production. Onions are what I always refer to as 'little collagen warriors' - they not only deliver high levels of sulphur to the body, they are also a good source of vitamin C, which helps to build and maintain our collagen levels.

Finally, here are 10 things (in no particular order) that contribute to skin stress and prematurely age the skin.

1. Excess alcohol
2. Mental anxiety
3. Smoking and drugs
4. Low exercise
5. Saturated fats
6. Excessive sun exposure
7. Polluted air
8. Not enough sleep
9. Excess weight
10. Sugar consumption

# 5-DAY SKIN DETOX CLEANSE

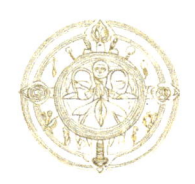

*Food is more than just taste; it can create deep therapeutic changes that heal, energise and nourish the body and the skin.*

**A healthy diet is what supports your face to look healthy and vital. What we put on the inside, shows up on the outside.**

This is why the stress we feel, along with environmental stressors (sun, pollution etc.) and lifestyle toxins in the form of fast food, alcohol and smoking all create skin stress which ages the skin.

This cleanse has been created to counteract skin stress and support your body's natural ability to eliminate and neutralise toxins. This enables the skin to heal naturally and function at its best.

Very quickly you will find your face loses excess fluid and puffiness, fine lines will be less apparent, skin will feel firmer and the skin will start to regain its natural glow.

This detox cleanse includes a high daily intake of parsley. The reason for this is that parsley is a superfood for skin. It has three times as much Vitamin C as oranges and twice as much iron as spinach, and it is also rich in Vitamins A and K, zinc, potassium and copper; which are all vital in the process of building and protecting your skin's collagen.

I recommend following this eating program for five days and then incorporating some of the key elements into your lifestyle. This will continue to support your skin to counteract skin stress and age less, which over time will help to stop premature aging and keep your skin looking more youthful and vital.

**Important:** Remember to drink at least 8 glasses of water each day in addition to the parsley tea to support toxin release.

You will see that there are no set amounts for most of the ingredients in these recipes. That is because their success doesn't rely on specific measurements, but the use of all ingredients in moderation. Remember it isn't a diet for losing weight, (although you might), this eating plan is all about supporting the detoxification and overall health of your skin.

So if you would like a little extra olive oil, ginger, chilli or any other ingredient, it is up to you.

**Tip:** Use herbs instead of salt to enhance the flavour of your cooking.

**Suggestion:** If you don't like salmon, you can substitute it for an oily fish such as sardines, tuna or mackerel. If you don't eat fish, you can substitute the salmon for tofu. Tofu contains the anti-oxidant genistein that is known to support skin elasticity.

## COOKING THE SALMON

To steam the salmon place a steamer rack in a closed pot over water. Once the water, (which can be infused with herbs for flavour) has reached boiling point, carefully place the salmon in the steam rack and cook for 5-6 minutes until pale orange in colour.

## MAKING THE PARSLEY TEA

**To make the tea you will need:**

- An infuser and teapot
- Half a cup of flat or curly leaf parsley roughly chopped and placed into the infuser
- Boiling water to fill the teapot

Steep tea for at least 10 minutes

**Tip:** Parsley tea can be served hot, warm or cold. To change the flavour add a little honey or lemon juice. It can be stored in the refrigerator for up to two days.

## THE IMPORTANCE OF WATER

Water is a vital element to maintaining plump, healthy looking skin, given that collagen (the skin's building block), is made up of approximately 60% water.

We need a minimum of eight glasses of water a day to flush out and eliminate toxins and purify the body. Consider adding lemon to your water as it not only cleanses the body, it contains vitamin C, which supports collagen production and elasticity (firmness) of the skin.

**Best times to drink water...**

**In the morning:** Have two glasses of semi-warm water on waking. It works as a natural detox for the body and helps rid the body of toxins and free radicals that have accumulated overnight.

**When hungry:** Often when we are hungry we are just thirsty and feeling de-hydrated. So before you snack on something, slowly drink a large glass of water and see how you feel in 10 minutes.

**When feeling tired:** Fatigue is one of the signs of dehydration, so when you are feeling tired, drink a glass of water to hydrate the brain and support increased cognitive function.

**When you exercise:** Drink water before and after you exercise to ensure you don't dehydrate and stress the body.

**When you bath:** Drink water before and after a bath.

**When you go to bed:** Drink water before bed to keep the body hydrated.

# MONDAY

*Your beauty is like a fire deep within you waiting to be lit. Don't wait, get in there and light it.*

## BREAKFAST

1 cup of boiled water with half a fresh lemon squeezed into it
2 egg white omelette, handful of baby spinach and a pinch of cumin
Do not add salt
1 serve of fruit
1-2 cups of parsley tea

## LUNCH

1 small can of tuna mixed with 1 chopped tomato, half a cucumber and a handful of spinach leaves, topped with walnuts and fresh parsley
Squeeze half a fresh lemon and a teaspoon of olive oil over the salad
*Optional:* add some cumin and chilli to the salad dressing
2 cups of parsley tea

## DINNER

Steamed salmon fillet with a mixed salad garnished with fresh parsley
1 cup of parsley tea
*Optional:* make a mixture of curry powder, cumin, ginger, garlic and a tablespoon of olive oil as a paste for coating the salmon

## SNACK

Handful of sunflower seeds

**Green juice:**
2 green apples, 2 cups of spinach and ½ a cup of parsley

Process ingredients together in a juicer. This juice is loaded with Vitamins A, K, B and C, iron and the antioxidant lutein.

## TUESDAY
*Pray daily, sing regularly, dance freely and meditate. It is the exercise that keeps your heart and soul defined.*

## BREAKFAST
1 cup of boiled water with half a fresh lemon squeezed into it
1 cup of low fat yoghurt with some strawberries and an apple or pear chopped up and mixed in
1-2 cups of parsley tea

## LUNCH
1 small tin of sardines with tomato, cucumber and lettuce, finished with fresh lemon juice and fresh parsley
*Optional:* add chilli or cumin to the lemon dressing
1 serve of fruit
2 cups of parsley tea

## DINNER
Steamed salmon fillet. Pan fry mushrooms, 1 zucchini and four cloves of garlic and serve on a bed of spinach
Season with fresh lemon juice, a teaspoon of virgin olive oil, ginger, fresh parsley and fresh mint (optional)
1 cup of parsley tea

## SNACK
Handful of sunflower seeds

**Green juice:**
2 green apples, 2 cups of spinach and ½ a cup of parsley processed together in a juicer.

## WEDNESDAY

*The world is only complete and beautiful when we recognise our own and know we have a place in it.*

### BREAKFAST
1 cup of boiled water with half a fresh lemon squeezed into it
1 cup of unflavoured oatmeal with a sliced pear
1-2 cups of parsley tea

### LUNCH
1 small tin of salmon on lettuce, tomato and parsley salad, dressed with 1 teaspoon of lemon juice and olive oil
*Optional:* add chilli, cumin and turmeric to the salad dressing
1 piece of melon, an apple or a pear
1-2 cups of parsley tea

### DINNER
Steamed salmon fillet with assorted vegetables - zucchini, broccoli and cauliflower
Season with fresh parsley, a teaspoon of olive oil and lemon, a pinch of cumin and some black pepper
1 cup of parsley tea

### SNACK
Handful of sunflower seeds

**Green juice:**
2 green apples, 2 cups of spinach and ½ a cup of parsley processed together in a juicer.

## THURSDAY

*The beauty we search for outside ourselves is a small aspect of what lies within. If you don't go within you will always go without.*

### BREAKFAST
1 cup of boiled water with half a fresh lemon squeezed into it
2 egg white omelette with spinach and chopped parsley
1 piece of fresh fruit
1-2 cups of parsley tea

### LUNCH
1 small tin of tuna or sardines and half a cup of bean salad
*Optional:* add parsley, chilli and/or ginger to the bean salad
1 piece of fresh fruit
2 cups of parsley tea

### DINNER
Steamed salmon fillet with steamed asparagus, green beans, garlic and zucchini, seasoned with fresh parsley, ginger and olive oil
1 cup of parsley tea

### SNACK
Handful of sunflower seeds

**Green juice:**
2 green apples, 2 cups of spinach and ½ a cup of parsley processed together in a juicer.

## FRIDAY

*We have the ability to enhance the beauty in our lives; all it takes is a willingness to let go of any thoughts, words and deeds that no longer support us.*

### BREAKFAST
1 cup of boiled water with half a fresh lemon squeezed into it
1 cup of unflavoured oatmeal with a sliced banana
1-2 cups of parsley tea

### LUNCH
1 steamed salmon fillet with steamed green vegetables, seasoned with fresh parsley, lemon juice and virgin olive oil
1 piece of fresh fruit and 2 cups of parsley tea

### DINNER
Steamed salmon fillet
Sauce: Sauté 1 onion, 1 small tin tomatoes, chopped capsicum, zucchini and a clove of garlic
Season with lemon juice, olive oil and fresh parsley
1 piece of fresh fruit and 1 cup of parsley tea

### SNACK
Handful of sunflower seeds

**Green juice:**
2 green apples, 2 cups of spinach and ½ a cup of parsley processed together in a juicer.

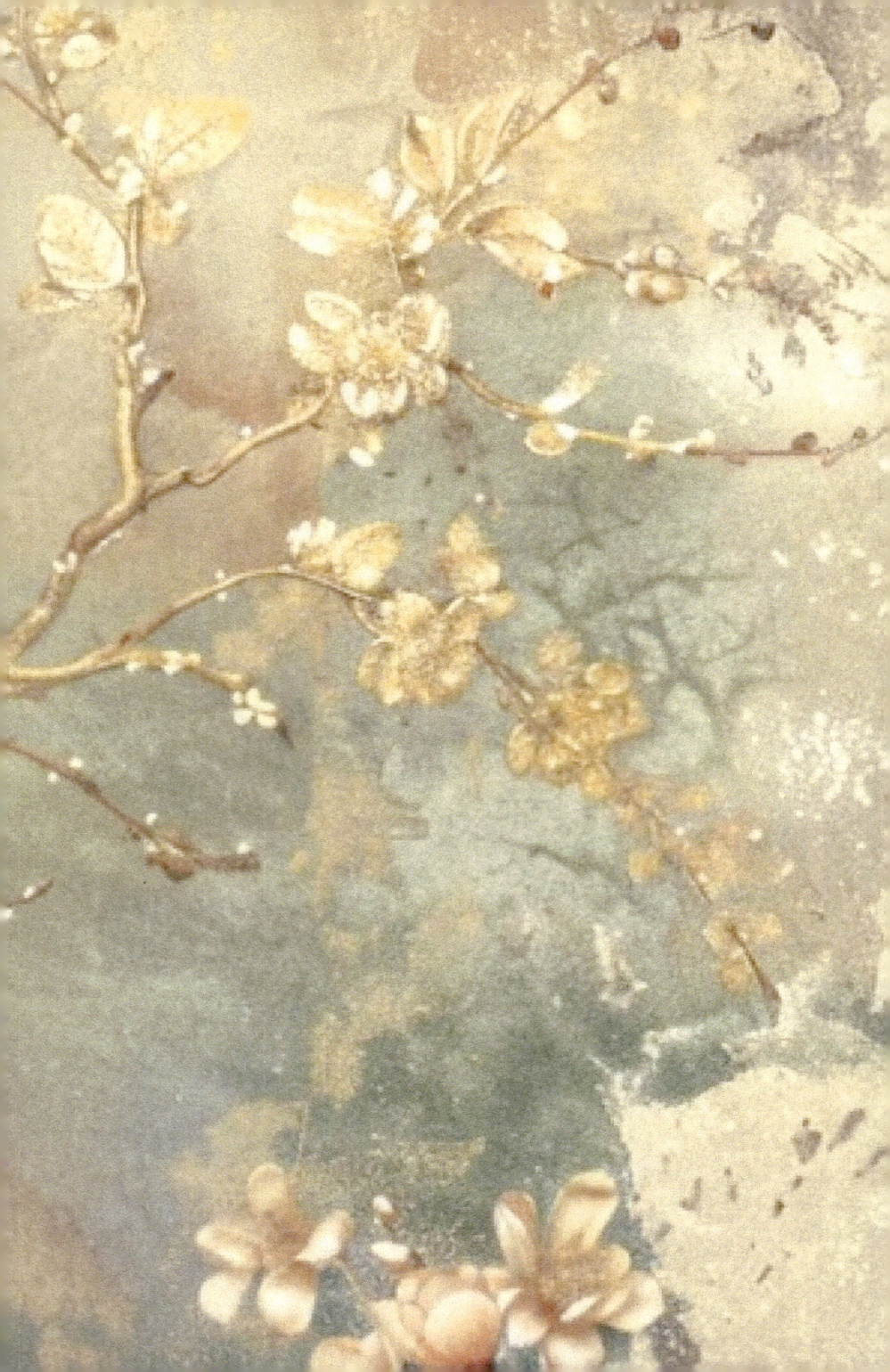

# FACE LIFTING FOOD BREAKFAST OPTIONS

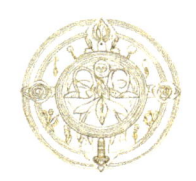

1. Collagen Building Smoothies
2. Skin Rejuvenating Tossed Fruit
3. Antioxidant Hot Porridge
4. Skin Boosting Muesli
5. Anti-Inflammatory Egg Omelette
6. Radiant Skin Watermelon Mix
7. Skin Moisturising Avocado On Wholegrain Toast
8. Skin Strengthening Berry & Yoghurt Mix

# COLLAGEN BUILDING SMOOTHIE

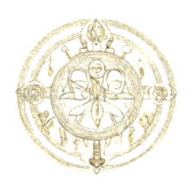

*The hidden power of beauty unfolds when we acknowledge that we are born with it.*

- Pour 350ml of pineapple or orange juice in a blender.
- Add around 130g of chopped fresh fruit such as bananas, strawberries, peaches, nectarines, mango or apricots.
- Add 2-3 tbsp natural low-fat yoghurt and blend.

THE SKIN SECRET:

**Citrus juice** – *Vitamin C (collagen building)* and **low-fat yoghurt** – *Vitamin A (regenerative)* protects and stabilises collagen.

# SKIN REJUVENATING TOSSED FRUIT

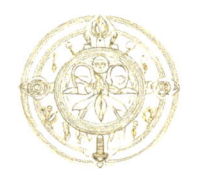

*To recognise our beauty as an individual is the ultimate potential that connects us to others and the world in a healthy way*

- Chop at least three different fruits into small pieces and mix together.
- Top with natural low-fat yoghurt.
- A teaspoon of honey is optional.

THE SKIN SECRET:

**Fruit** – *Vitamin C (collagen building);* **natural yoghurt** – *Vitamin A (anti-aging); and* **honey** – *antioxidant,* are collagen and elastin building which keep the skin strong, smooth and firm, while increasing elasticity.

SKIN REMINDER:

**Banana** - the antioxidants and nutrients in bananas help to restore collagen in your skin. They also have antibacterial properties and can be applied to the face mashed with lemon (stops the banana going brown) or with yoghurt, honey, egg or milk for a range of benefits that assist in maintaining the health of the skin.

# ANTIOXIDANT HOT PORRIDGE

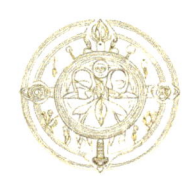

*Beauty reflects our true self*

- Make oats according to the instructions on the packet and add skim milk, skim soy or oat milk.
- *Optional:* add honey, chopped dates or sultanas.
- Sprinkle with shaved almonds.

THE SKIN SECRET:
*Oats – Vitamin A, selenium and magnesium and* **almonds –** *Vitamin E and Potassium* are high in antioxidants and improve circulation and skin moisture retention.

# SKIN BOOSTING MUESLI

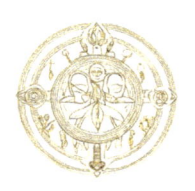

*To recognise the beauty in the world we must recognise the beauty in ourselves*

- Make your muesli from your favourite sugarless grains or purchase a natural muesli that is predominantly grains.
- Add prunes to your taste, sunflower seeds and pumpkin seeds.
- Serve with soy milk or orange juice and top with natural yoghurt and linseeds.
- Add whatever fresh fruit you have on hand chopped finely.

THE SKIN SECRET:

**Oats** – *Vitamin A (anti-aging), selenium and magnesium;* **prunes** – *Vitamins A and C (collagen building) and Potassium;* **sunflower** *and* **pumpkin seeds** – *Vitamin E, Selenium, Copper; Omega-3 and*

*Niacin; and* **natural yoghurt** *– Vitamin A* build collagen and the rich antioxidant mix gives skin a healthy, dewy glow.

SKIN REMINDER:

**Prunes** - contain one of the highest levels of antioxidants (Blueberries are a close runner up). Eat five to seven prunes for a skin boost.

# ANTI-INFLAMMATORY EGG OMELETTE

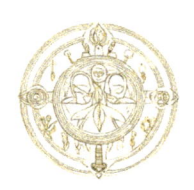

*Beauty is a process that opens us up to*
*liberate the mind and uplift the soul*

2 egg whites, 1 whole egg (or 3 egg whites in total) with a handful of spinach

*Optional:* Parsley and Spring onions

- Beat the eggs together while bringing a non-stick medium sized frying pan to moderate heat.
- Pour in the mixture and swirl to ensure full coverage of the pan.
- After 30 seconds add spinach (and finely chopped parsley and spring onions).
- When egg on the inside of the omelette is no longer liquid, fold one side over the other to create a pasty shape using a spatular.
- Sprinkle with small amount of sea salt or Parmesan if required.

THE SKIN SECRET:

*Eggs* – *Vitamins A (skin building) and D, and* **Spinach** – *Vitamin A, C, E and K with anti-inflammatory antioxidants* **improve the texture and tone of the skin.**

# RADIANT SKIN WATERMELON REFRESHER

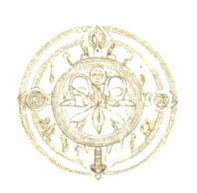

*The awareness of living moment to moment has a profound force of awakening our beauty*

Roughly chop up watermelon (desired amount) into a bowl and add low-fat yoghurt and mint or enjoy plain.

THE SKIN SECRET:

**Watermelon** – *strong antioxidant with Vitamins A (skin renewing), B and C (collagen building);* **Low-fat yoghurt** – *Vitamin A; and* **Mint** – *Vitamin C* **stimulate the skin's own age protective antioxidants.**

SKIN REMINDER:

**Watermelon** is high in the super antioxidant lycopene and Vitamins A, B and C (collagen building), which keep the skin fresh, radiant and hydrated. The natural acids can also act as an exfoliant, which when applied topically can be used to reduce blemishes.

# SKIN MOISTURISING AVOCADO ON WHOLEGRAIN TOAST

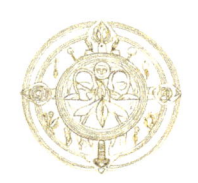

*Nutritious food is one of the best beauty treatments anyone can give themselves*

Half a ripe avocado

1 slice of thickly cut wholegrain bread (spelt, rye, stone ground wholemeal)

- Toast the bread and add slices of avocado.
- Garnish with parsley and a sprinkle of sea salt (optional)

**Note:** *A spread such as home made relish or mustard can be used to flavour the toast before adding the avocado.*

THE SKIN SECRET:

*Avocado – Vitamins E and K and* **Wholegrain bread** *– Vitamin B complex, Selenium, Copper and Phosphorus* **reduce fine lines,**

**deeply moisturise and enhance the overall tone of your skin.**

SKIN REMINDER:

**Avocado** used topically tightens the skin and penetrates the layers to the deepest level. It is good for reducing fine lines and enhancing overall skin tone. Avocado contains more than 25 essential nutrients and Vitamins including Vitamins E and K.

# SKIN STRENGTHENING BERRY & YOGURT MIX

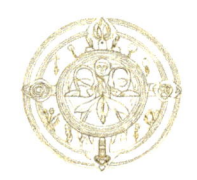

*It is in those quiet reflective moments
that we recognise our beauty*

Mix frozen berries (any) with natural low-fat yoghurt (honey is optional) and enjoy as a whole breakfast or add to your low sugar cereal or muesli.

THE SKIN SECRET:

**Berries** – *strong antioxidants full of Vitamins A (skin smoothing) and C (collagen building), Potassium and Calcium and* **Low-fat yoghurt** *with Vitamin A* **build collagen and elastin while strengthening the underlying skin structure.**

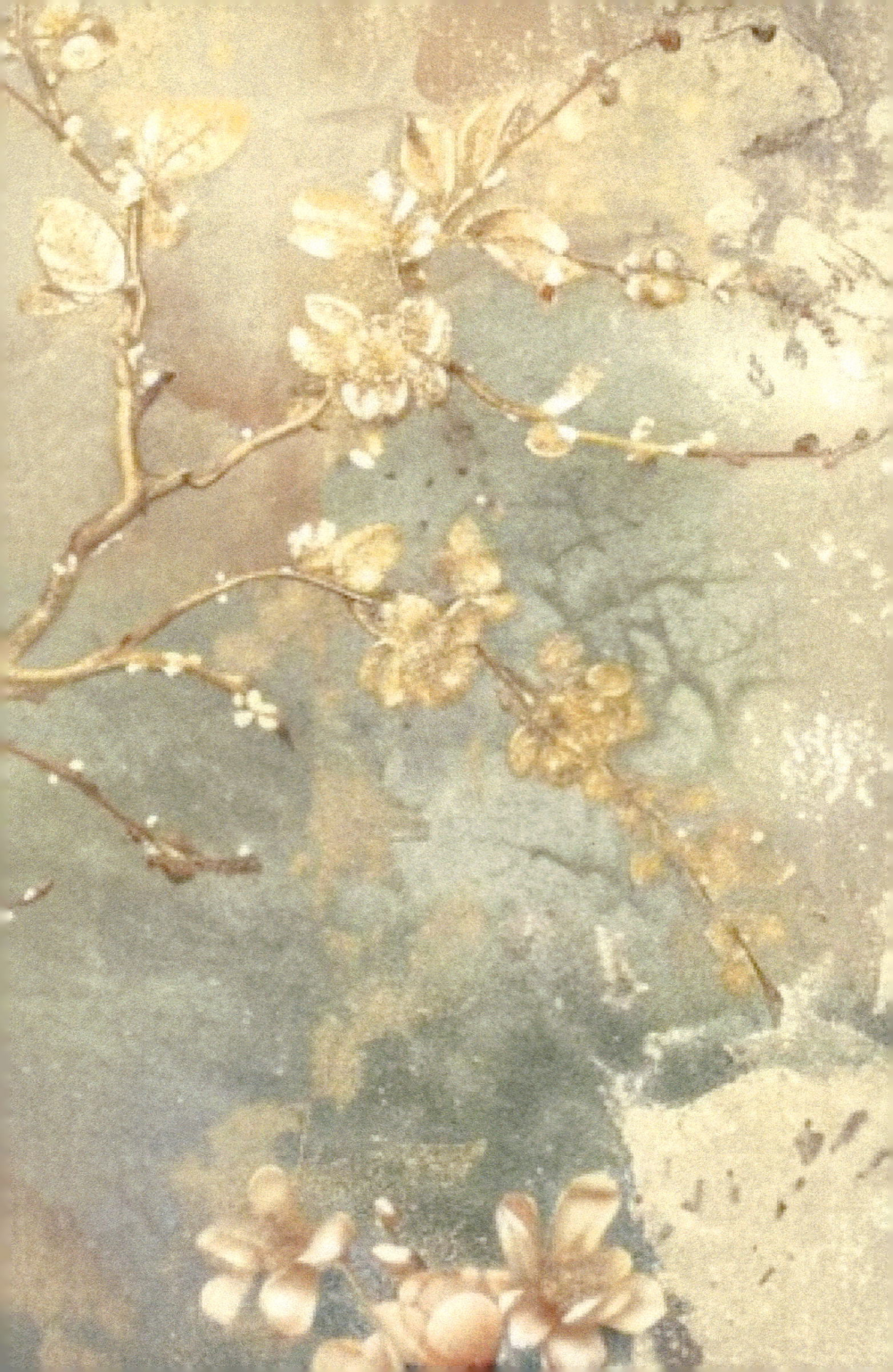

# FACE LIFTING FOOD LUNCH OPTIONS

1. Skin Plumping Sardine Bruschetta
2. Vitamin E Loaded Salad Dressing
3. Calcium Rich Veggie Frittata
4. Potassium Filled Tuna Potatoes
5. Vitamin A Skin Renewing Smoked Trout Salad
6. A & C Skin Building Pea Soup
7. Collagen Corn and Pepper Soup
8. 'C' Bean Salad
9. Potassium Packed Spanish Salad
10. Skin Rebuilding Spiced Cauliflower
11. Nurturing Antioxidant Avocado Citrus Salad

# SKIN PLUMPING SARDINE BRUSCHETTA

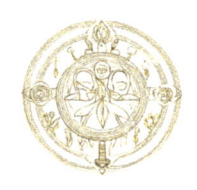

*Food is what we make it*
*Our skin is what we feed it*

2 tins of sardines (in fresh water)
1 (400g) tin of peeled tomatoes
2 cloves of garlic (optional)
Finely chopped red onion
1 tbsp Dijon mustard (optional)
1 tbsp olive oil
Wholegrain bread rolls
Handful of finely chopped fresh basil or parsley

- Place the half cut rolls in a hot oven for 2 minutes.
- Mix the tomatoes, onion, garlic, mustard and olive oil in a bowl and season with pepper, chilli or herbs of your choice.
- Remove rolls and spoon over mixture.

- Place sardines on top and return to the oven for 3 minutes.
- Serve warm with an additional drizzle of olive oil over the top.
- Alternatively serve mixture on rice crackers without heating.

THE SKIN SECRET:

***Sardines*** *– Omega 3, Coenzyme Q10, Calcium, Selenium, Vitamins B and D;* **Tomato** *– Potassium, Vitamins A (skin regenerating) and C (collagen building);* **Garlic** *– Vitamin C and Selenium and* **Wholegrain rolls** *– Vitamin B complex, Selenium, Copper and Phosphorus* **plump up the skin with essential fatty acids and reduce fine lines.**

SKIN REMINDER:

Sardines are a wonderful source of Omega-3 fatty acids, which are responsible for healthy skin membranes – moisturising the skin and improving its texture and softness. Sardines also contain Coenzyme Q10 a powerful anti-aging antioxidant.

# VITAMIN E LOADED SALAD DRESSING

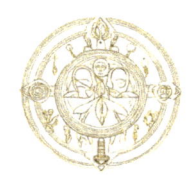

*We build our beauty and our deepest sense of self worth when we focus on our strengths instead of our weaknesses*

To serve with any side serving of greens...

2 tbsp olive oil
1 tbsp balsamic vinegar
1 clove of garlic
Pinch of sea salt
Pinch of black pepper

THE SKIN SECRET:

**Olive oil** – *antioxidant full of Vitamins E and K and* **Garlic** – *strong antioxidant high in Vitamin C (collagen building) and K* **support elasticity and add to skin lustre.**

SKIN REMINDER:

**Olive Oil** is an antioxidant high in Vitamin E and Vitamin K (found in green leafy vegetables), and contains high antioxidant and anti- inflammatory properties that help counteract exposure to pollution, smoke, alcohol and other damaging free radicals. Olive oil is so rich in its nutrient value that it can be used topically on any part of the body to moisturise and regenerate. Vitamin E also helps regulate the presence of Vitamin A in the body, essential for healthy skin.

# CALCIUM RICH VEGGIE FRITTATA

*Every positive thought we have has the capacity to enrich our beauty and our lives*

4 eggs
1 tbsp milk
1 cup of your favourite chopped vegetables (such as peppers, mushrooms, carrots, broccoli, pumpkin)
Olive oil spray

- Preheat the oven to a medium heat.
- Chop the vegetables finely.
- Mix beaten eggs in a bowl with pepper or other flavourings (fresh thyme, basil, chilli, curry powder or black pepper).
- Stir fry the veg for 2-3 minutes in a non stick pan that has been sprayed with olive oil spray.
- Pour the egg mixture into the pan and cook for 4-5

minutes until the mixture is setting on both the top and bottom.
- Place pan in the oven and cook for 4-5 minutes or until lightly browned.
- Remove from heat and serve.

THE SKIN SECRET:

*Eggs - Vitamins A (skin building) and D; Milk - Vitamins A and D as well as minerals Calcium, Phosphorous, Potassium, Selenium, Magnesium and Zinc; and Veg – Potassium, Vitamins A and C (collagen building)* **increase the skin's elasticity and are full of antioxidants and skin building minerals.**

SKIN REMINDER:

**Eggs** contain Vitamins A, D, Niacin, Phosphorus, Selenium and proteins. When applied topically eggs have a tightening and constricting effect on the pores and egg whites used as a mask will remove dead skin cells.

# POTASSIUM FILLED TUNA POTATOES

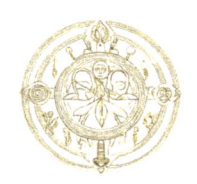

*You are never too old or too young to make a difference to your skin*

500g small potatoes (in their skins)
1 large tin of tuna
1 tin of sliced mushrooms (champignons)
3 spring onions (chopped)
3 tbsp chopped chives
Handful of green beans
Ground pepper or chilli to taste
4 tbsp natural low-fat yoghurt

- Cook potatoes in boiling water for five minutes or until tender. Drain and leave to cook for five minutes before breaking the tops gently.
- Mix tuna, spring onions, mushrooms and beans and serve on a plate.

- Mix chives and yoghurt and spoon over the top of the opened potatoes.
- Season with black pepper or chilli.

THE SKIN SECRET:

*Tuna – Omega-3, Niacin, Selenium, Magnesium and Potassium; Potatoes – Vitamin C (collagen building), Potassium and Zinc; Green beans – Potassium, Phosphorus and Zinc; and Yoghurt - Vitamin A* **repair the skin while building collagen.**

SKIN REMINDER:

**Yoghurt** is high in Alpha Hydroxy Acid (skin renewal), Vitamins A and B5 and when applied topically will act as a gentle exfoliant that increases the moisture content in skin and hair. It will also cool and soothe irritated skin.

# VITAMIN A SKIN RENEWING SMOKED TROUT SALAD

*Once you have the motivation to eat well you will feel well and if you let it that feeling will guide you in every area of your life*

**Salad**
750g warm smoked trout 200g
Spinach leaves
2 medium peaches cut into small wedges
**Dressing**
Squeeze of lemon juice
1 tsp honey
1 tbsp yoghurt

- Mix ingredients for the dressing and set aside.
- Discard bones and skin from the trout, break into large pieces in a salad bowl, add spinach and peaches then mix gently.
- Serve with salad dressing.

THE SKIN SECRET:

*Trout* – *Vitamin A (skin rebuilding), Omega-3, selenium and calcium;* **Spinach** – *Vitamins A, C (collagen building), E and K;* **Peaches** – *Vitamins A, E and K;* **Low-fat yoghurt** – *Vitamin A;* and **Lemon juice** – *Vitamin C, Potassium and Calcium* **rebuilds and strengthens collagen while Omega 3 makes skin glow.**

SKIN REMINDER:

**Peaches** are a great source of antioxidants which help protect your skin from UV rays. Research has shown that nutrients from topically applied juice benefit the strength and elasticity of skin.

# A & C SKIN BUILDING PEA SOUP

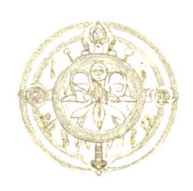

*We have the power to create our own beauty destiny by the way we choose to live and love*

1 tbsp olive oil
1 small onion (chopped)
3 spring onions (chopped)
2 cups fresh or frozen peas
¼ cup low-fat natural yoghurt
1 cup chicken stock ( low salt stock cubes or liquid)
¼ cup fresh mint or parsley
1 tbsp fresh ginger (very finely chopped)
Seasonings to taste (pepper, chilli, turmeric)

- Heat the oil in a large pot.
- Sauté the onion and spring onions until clear.
- Add peas, ginger and chicken stock and simmer until peas are tender.
- Add mint and seasonings to taste.

- Remove from heat and leave to cool until it can be blended in a food processor.
- Heat and serve with a spoon of low-fat yoghurt.

THE SKIN SECRET:

***Onion*** *– Vitamin C (collagen building);* ***Peas*** *– Vitamins A (skin regenerating), C and K with zinc and Potassium;* ***Low-fat yoghurt*** *– Vitamin A; and Parsley – Vitamins A, C and K* **give your skin a strong boost of Vitamins A and C together with skin repairing Zinc and Potassium for a healthy glow.**

SKIN REMINDER:

**Ginger** is known to be good for digestion and calming the stomach, but it is also an anti-inflammatory. It can also be applied topically to the skin to great effect.

## COLLAGEN CORN AND PEPPER SOUP

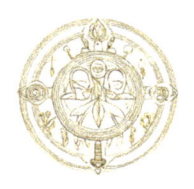

*If you want to see lasting changes in your skin then make lasting changes to your diet*

600g jar of roasted red peppers
1 cup chicken stock ( from low salt stock cubes or liquid)
300ml natural yoghurt (reserve 50g to add when serving)
1 tsp curry powder
350ml low-fat soy milk
2 cups cooked corn kernels

- Blend all ingredients (except the corn) in a food processor and pour into a medium pan.
- Add corn and simmer for 6 minutes.
- Serve with natural yoghurt.

THE SKIN SECRET:

*Red peppers* – *Vitamin C (collagen building);* **Corn kernels** – *Vitamin B complex (including Niacin);* **Natural Yoghurt** – *Vitamin A (skin renewing); and* **Curry spices** – *antioxidants* **build collagen and feed your body powerful antioxidants to protect the skin.**

# 'C' BEAN SALAD

*Skin is like life, you only get out
of it what you put in*

## Salad
2 cups cooked red beans drained (canned or fresh)
1 garlic clove (chopped)
¼ cup onion (finely chopped)
½ cup green capsicum (finely chopped)
¼ cup coriander or parsley
1 tbsp sweet chilli sauce
1 tsp ground cumin or turmeric (optional)

## Dressing
120ml olive oil
3 tbsp lemon juice
Mix salad together in a large bowl and add dressing to serve.

THE SKIN SECRET:

*Red Beans – Copper, Potassium and Zinc;* **Garlic** *– Vitamin C, Selenium;* **Green Capsicum** *– Vitamin C (collagen building);* **Onion** *– Vitamin C;* **Parsley** *- Vitamins A (skin building) and C; and* **Spice** *antioxidants* **nurture skin with essential minerals to build collagen and elastin.**

SKIN REMINDER:

**Parsley** has three times as much Vitamin C as oranges and twice as much iron as spinach. It is also rich in Vitamins A and K and Potassium, which together build collagen and help strengthen the connective tissue of skin. Parsley is high in Vitamins A and K and can be applied topically to reduce dark under eye circles.

# POTASSIUM PACKED SPANISH SALAD

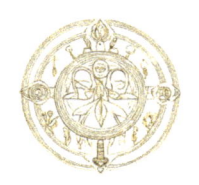

*Beauty is not a secret, it is a revelation*

## Salad
4 cups mixed leafy salad torn into pieces
½ cup red or green onion
1 tomato (sliced)
¼ cup black olives (pitted)
2 artichoke hearts (cut in quarters)
1 tsp fresh herbs (basil, rosemary, parsley)

## Dressing
1 tbsp extra virgin olive oil
1 tbsp lemon juice
1 tbsp balsamic vinegar
1 tsp Dijon mustard

- Mix the dressing ingredients together until well

combined and pour over the prepared salad ingredients. Toss and serve.

THE SKIN SECRET:

*Leafy greens* – *Vitamin C (collagen building) and Potassium;* *Artichoke hearts* – *Vitamin C, Potassium and Magnesium ;* *Olive oil* – *Vitamins E and K;* *Tomato* – *Vitamins A (skin regenerating) and C and Potassium;* *Lemon juice* – *Vitamin C, Calcium and Potassium; and* *Basil* – *Vitamins A and C, and Beta carotene* **hydrate and boost the skin.**

SKIN REMINDER:

**Tomatoes** are high in Vitamins A and C and the antioxidant Lycopene which helps even out skin pigmentation when applied topically.

# SKIN BUILDING SPICED CAULIFLOWER

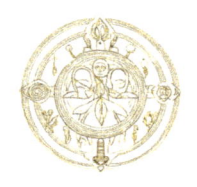

*The cornerstone to beautiful skin is beautiful food*

3 tbsp olive oil
1 tsp cumin seeds
2 cm fresh ginger
¼ tsp each of Indian spices - ground coriander, cayenne, turmeric, garam masala (any or all)
1 medium onion
1 tomato (diced)
1 medium cauliflower (cut into small florets)
1 large potato (cubed)
1 cup frozen peas
½ cup water
Sliced fresh green chilli (optional)

- Heat oil in a large pan and toast the cumin seeds.
- Add garlic, chilli and ginger and sauté for 2 minutes.

- Add onion and tomato and sauté for 3 minutes.
- Stir in the Indian spices
- Add the potato, cauliflower and water and cook for 10 minutes.
- Add peas and ¼ cup of water and cook for further 7 minutes until water has evaporated and vegetable are soft.

THE SKIN SECRET:

**Cauliflower** – *Vitamins C and K, Potassium and Niacin;* **Ginger** – *Zinc;* **Indian spices** – *antioxidants;* **Peas** – *Vitamins A (skin regenerating) and C, Zinc and Potassium; and* **Potato** – *Vitamin C, Potassium and Zinc* **build the strength of the skin.**

SKIN REMINDER:

**Cauliflower** is high in Selenium and contains Vitamins A and C, together with Niacin, Phosphorous and Calcium.

# NURTURING ANTIOXIDANT AVOCADO CITRUS SALAD

*Beauty is expressed with kindness, nurtured with love and strengthened with self belief*

4 cups mixed greens
1 ripe avocado
1 cup orange or grapefruit segments (cut into ¼ segments) 1 small red pepper (sliced into strips)
2 tbsp Basic Salad Dressing (see recipe)
Handful of peanuts to garnish

- Layer the greens, citrus segments, red pepper and avocado on a plate.
- Pour a small amount of the dressing over the salad and serve.

THE SKIN SECRET:
*Avocado – 25 essential minerals and vitamins including Vitamins E and K;* **Mixed greens** *– Vitamin C and Potassium;* **Citrus fruit** *– Vitamin C (collagen building);* **Peanuts** *– strong antioxidant; and* **Red pepper** *– Vitamin C and K* **nourish skin and stimulate collagen production.**

SKIN REMINDER:
**Peanuts** contain Oleic acid, the healthful fat in olive oil, but they are also rich in antioxidants – richer in fact than apples, carrots or beets.

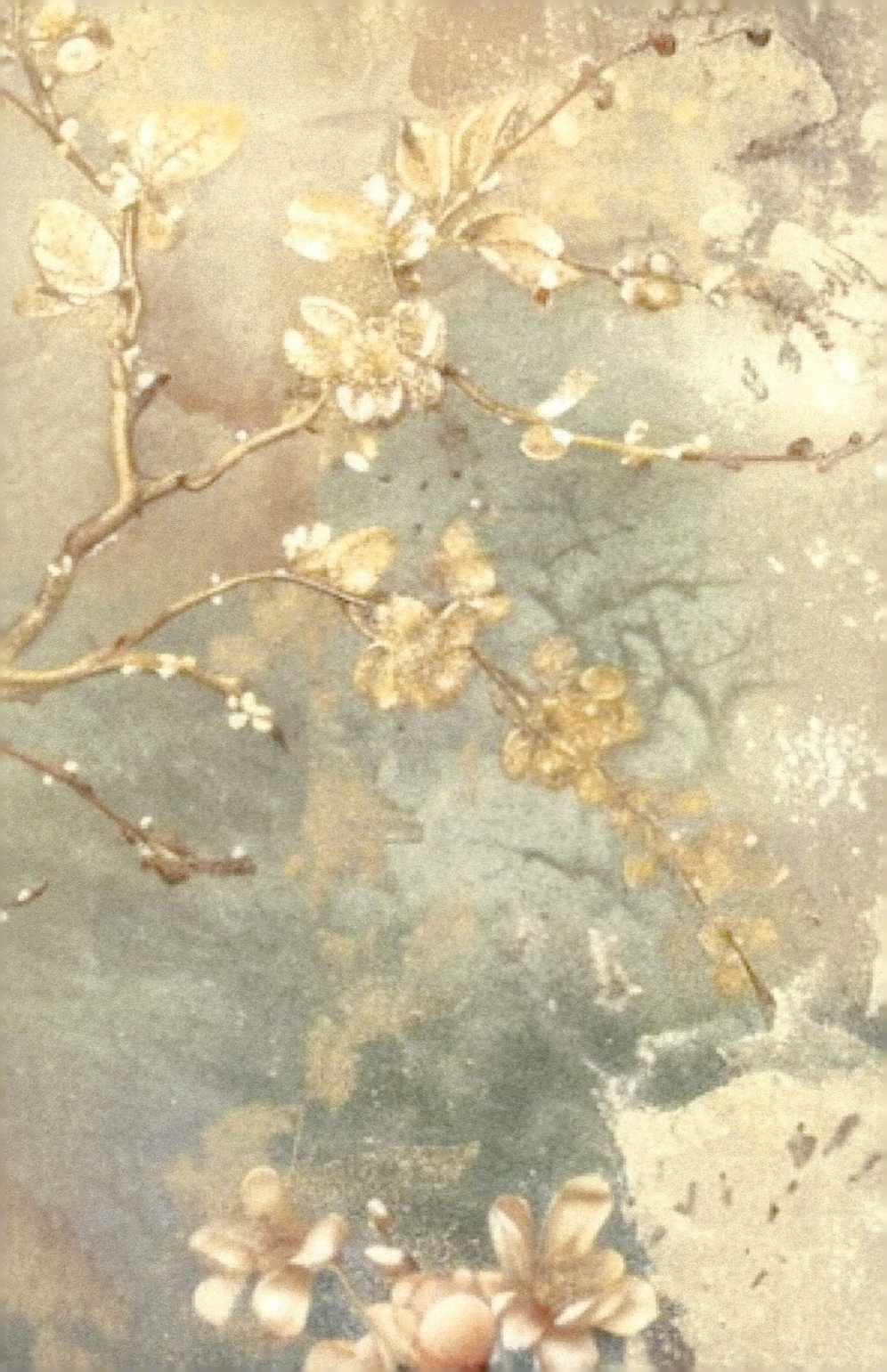

# FACE LIFTING FOOD DINNER OPTIONS

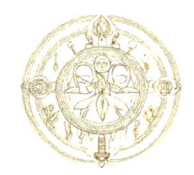

1. Skin Illuminating Mackerel With Salad
2. Collagen Building Poached Fish (Or Chicken)
3. Skin Protecting Chicken With Vegetables
4. Super Skin Antioxidant Salmon With Coconut
5. Antioxidant Salmon (Or Chicken) With Teriyaki Sauce
6. Wrinkle Prevention Fish (Or Chicken) Kebabs

# SKIN ILLUMINATING MACKEREL WITH SALAD

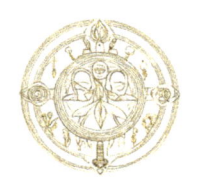

*Creativity is like beauty,
it loves individuality*

1 can of mackerel fillets (or fresh)
Olive oil (for brushing)
Black pepper or chilli

**Sauce**
200ml olive oil
1 tbsp of sweet chilli sauce
1 tbsp Worcestershire sauce
1 tsp parsley (chopped)
1 tsp rosemary (chopped)
3 tsp spring onion (chopped)
2 long green chillies (chopped, optional)
Spinach leaves and half a sliced
Continental cucumber to serve

- Mix olive oil, sweet chilli sauce and Worcestershire sauce and add all chopped ingredients.
- Sprinkle mackerel fillets with pepper or chilli and brush with olive oil.
- Pan fry (without oil in a non-stick pan) for 2 minutes either side and serve on a bed of spinach and cucumber.
- Dress with the sauce.

THE SKIN SECRET:

*Mackerel* – *Vitamin A (skin regenerating), Omega-3 and Omega-6;* **Rosemary** – *Beta carotene, Vitamins A, C (collagen building), E and K;* **Parsley** – *Vitamins A, C and K;* **Olive oil** – *Vitamins E and K; and* **Spinach** – *Beta carotene, Vitamins A, B, C, E and K* **plump up your skin and give it a natural radiance.**

SKIN REMINDER:

Cucumber - contains Vitamins A and C (collagen building) and is a strong antioxidant with a number of trace minerals and enzymes essential for skin growth and repair. It is a good source of silica, a trace mineral that contributes to the strength of connective tissue. Cucumber is immediately effective on puffy eyes, sunburn or as a tonic for the whole face.

# COLLAGEN BUILDING POACHED FISH (OR CHICKEN)

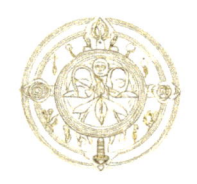

*The most beautiful person is usually the one who acknowledges that as human beings, we all have it*

4 fish fillets
Water
¼ cup white wine vinegar
4 sprigs fresh parsley
2 cloves fresh garlic
3 Bay leaves
Whole green peppercorns
1 tsp fennel seed or celery seeds

- Mix 1 tbsp low-fat yoghurt with 1 tsp capers (drained).
- Using a pan with a lid fill with approximately 2

centimetres of water, add all seasonings and bring to boil.
- Cover, reduce heat to low and simmer for about 10 minutes.
- Add fish, cover and simmer for approximately 5 minutes, turning once (depending on the thickness of the fish – when cooked it will be opaque and flaky).
- Can be served hot topped with the yoghurt caper sauce, a side of salad and lemon wedges; or served cold and taken as a lunch if prepared the night before.

THE SKIN SECRET:

***Fish** – Omega-3, Omega-6 and Vitamin A (skin regenerating);* ***Parsley** – Vitamins A, C (collagen building) and K;* ***Bay leaves** – Potassium, Vitamins A and C; and **Garlic** – Vitamin C and Selenium* **build collagen in the skin.**

SKIN REMINDER:

Tuna is an excellent source of Omega-3 fatty acid as well as being a good source of Potassium, Magnesium, Selenium, and Thiamin.

# SKIN PROTECTING CHICKEN WITH VEGETABLES

*Knowing our beauty is the centre of our wisdom*

1 tbsp extra virgin olive oil
750g skinless chicken breasts (cut into quarters) 300g Brussels sprouts
200g Yellow Squash
1½ cups chopped onion
2-3 tbsp fresh rosemary
1½ cups chicken stock (from low salt stock cubes or liquid)
Seasoning (black pepper, chilli) to taste

- Preheat oven to 190°C.
- In a pan heat the oil and brown the chicken.
- Place chicken in a shallow baking dish, sprinkle with onions and rosemary and season.
- Place the squash and the sprouts around the chicken and add the broth.
- Bake covered for 20 minutes.

- Uncover increasing the temperature to 210°C for a further 30-40 mins or until sprouts are cooked.
- Serve and enjoy!

THE SKIN SECRET:

***Skinless chicken*** – *Vitamin E, Zinc and Selenium;* ***Brussels sprouts*** – *Potassium, Vitamins A, C and K;* ***Yellow squash*** – *Vitamins A, C and K;* ***Rosemary*** – *Beta carotene, Vitamins A, C, E and K* **build collagen and improves texture of skin.**

SKIN REMINDER:

**Brussels sprouts** are extremely high in Vitamin C which is collagen building.

# SUPER SKIN ANTIOXIDANT SALMON WITH COCONUT

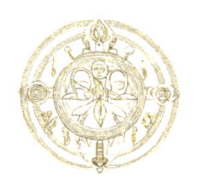

*Beauty makes room for everyone*

150g salmon fillets (skin removed)
1 tbsp lemon juice
½ cup dry breadcrumbs
¼ cup desiccated coconut
Season to taste (black pepper, chilli)
Olive oil cooking spray

- Preheat oven to 220°C. Place salmon fillets on a non-stick baking pan and brush with lemon juice.
- In a flat dish combine the breadcrumbs, coconut and seasoning.
- Coat each fillet with the mixture and spread left over crumbs on the top.
- Coat with olive oil cooking spray.
- Bake for 12-15 minutes and then place under the grill until the crust is golden brown.

- Serve with salad or oven baked vegetables.

## A COCONUT CHICKEN ALTERNATIVE

- A chicken alternative to this recipe is to roll strips of chicken breasts in natural yoghurt and then in the coconut and bread crumb mixture.
- Spray with cooking spray and bake in the oven at 230°C for 15 minutes and then a further 15 minutes at 180°C.

## THE SKIN SECRET:

*Salmon* – *DMAE, Niacin, Calcium, Zinc, Magnesium, Vitamins A and D;* *Lemon juice* – *Vitamin C, Calcium and Potassium* **improve the tone and texture of skin.**

## SKIN REMINDER:

**Tomatoes** are high in Vitamins A and C and the antioxidant Lycopene which helps even out skin pigmentation when applied topically.

# ANTIOXIDANT SALMON (OR CHICKEN) WITH TERIYAKI SAUCE

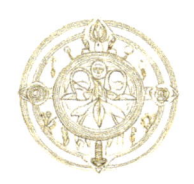

*As long as we remain open to people's differences we will always be surrounded by beauty*

Individual Salmon (or chicken) portions as required
1 bunch of Bok Choy per two persons (wash well)

**Sauce**
¼ cup soy sauce
1 cup orange juice
1 tbsp honey
1 tbsp chilli flakes (optional)
1 tsp grated ginger & 2 cloves fresh garlic

- Mix ingredients in a bowl.
- Place the salmon in a shallow dish and pour the sauce over the top, turning the fish at least once.
- Place fish on grease proof paper under the grill and

cook for 10-12 minutes (depending on the thickness and how well cooked you like it). Flip the fish once.
- When the salmon has one minute to go place broken up Bok Choy in a bowl with minimum water at the base covered with clear wrap for 1 minute. Serve salmon on a bed of the steamed Bok Choy.
- If using chicken fillets instead you will need to bake the chicken in the oven for 15 minutes before grilling for a further 10 minutes.

THE SKIN SECRET:

*Salmon – DMAE, Niacin, Calcium, Zinc, Magnesium, Vitamins A (skin regenerating) and D;* **Garlic** *– Vitamin C (collagen building) and Selenium;* **Honey** *– antioxidants;* **Ginger** *– Zinc;* **Orange Juice** *– Potassium, Vitamins A and C; and* **Bok Choy** *– Calcium, Potassium, Vitamins A, C and K* **deliver powerful antioxidants to the skin to assist with rebuilding fresh radiant skin.**

SKIN REMINDER:

**Citrus Fruits** contain Vitamin C (collagen building) which helps neutralise free radical activity and promote collagen synthesis – the key to skin remaining youthful and elastic. Juice can be applied to the face for an exfoliation treatment.

# WRINKLE PREVENTION FISH (OR CHICKEN) KEBABS

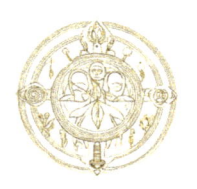

*What we eat is the ultimate skin hydration boost*

1 red pepper (cut into squares)
1 can of pineapple chunks
1 onion (cut into squares)
5 mushrooms (cut into chunks)
2 fish fillets or chicken breasts (cut into 2cm chunks)
Wooden skewers
Basting Sauce
¼ cup olive oil
2 tbsp balsamic vinegar
2 garlic cloves (crushed)
2 tsp honey
Seasoning to taste (sea salt, black pepper, chilli)

- Combine all the ingredients to make the basting sauce and toss the fish pieces in, mixing until covered.

- Arrange fish, peppers, mushrooms, onion and pineapple on skewers.
- Grill for around 12 minutes, basting the whole skewer and turning every 2 minutes until cooked (fish is opaque and chicken is white).

THE SKIN SECRET:

*Fish – Omega-3 and Vitamin A (skin regenerating);* **Pineapple** *– Vitamin C (collagen building);* **Red peppers** *– Vitamin C and K;* **Onion** *– Vitamin C;* **Garlic** *– Vitamin C and Selenium;* **Olive oil** *- Vitamin E and K; and* **Mushrooms** *– Potassium, Vitamins B (including Niacin) and D* **support the building of collagen while smoothing the skin and helping to prevent wrinkles.**

SKIN REMINDER:

To minimise its impact on collagen production sugar intake should be kept at a minimum, however it can be applied topically with water as a glycolic acid treatment.

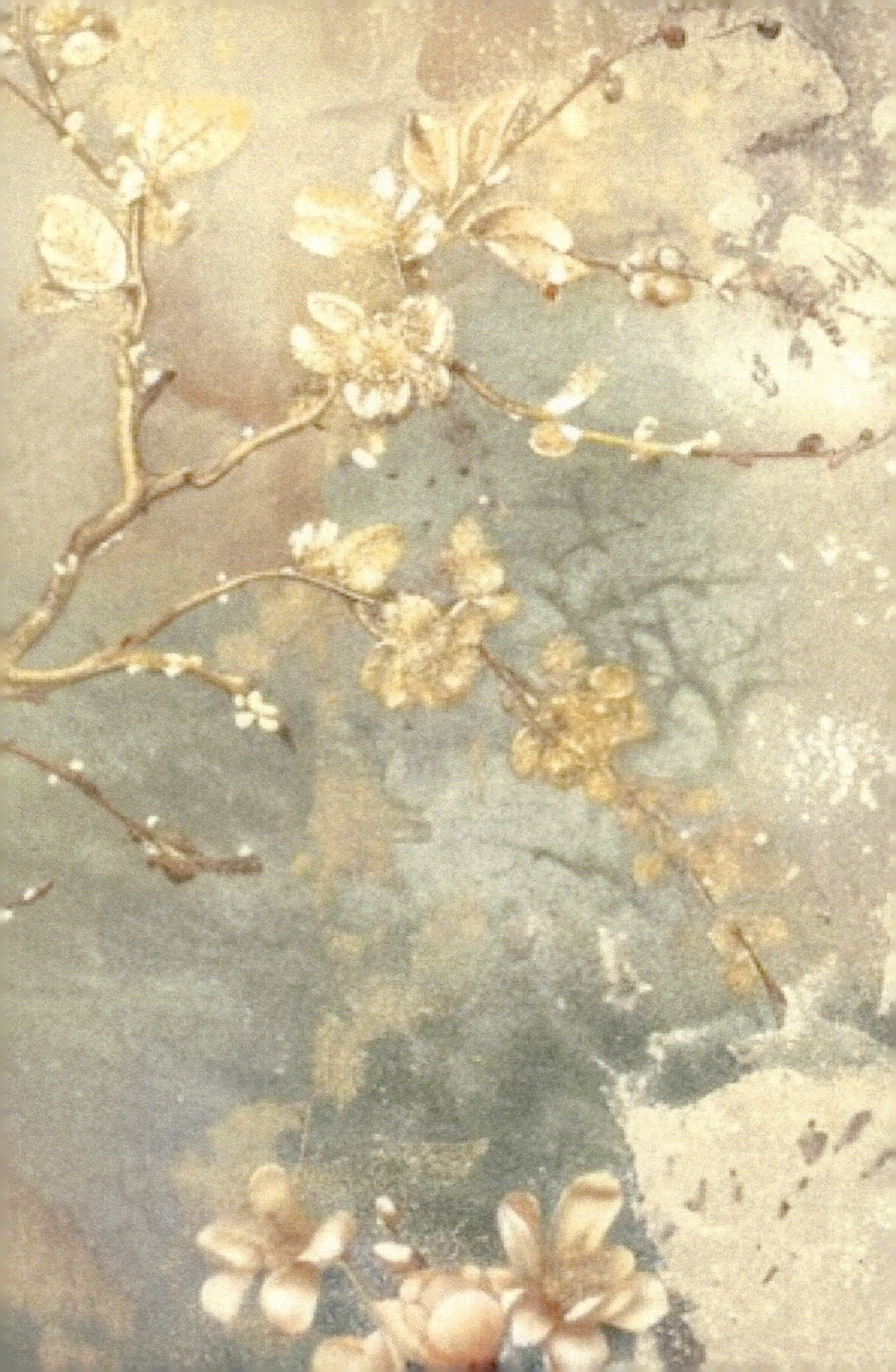

# FACE LIFTING FOOD SNACK OPTIONS

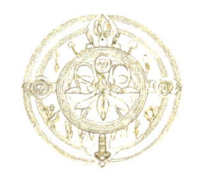

**1 cup of Natural Yoghurt mixed with berries**
THE SKIN SECRET: *Berries – Vitamins A (skin regenerating) and C (collagen building); and* **Yoghurt** *– Vitamin A,* **nurture your skin with Vitamins and essential minerals.**

**Handful of Almonds**
THE SKIN SECRET: *Almonds – Vitamin E and Potassium –* **give skin a healthy glow.**

**Celery and Carrot Sticks**
THE SKIN SECRET: *Celery – Vitamins A (skin rebuilding), C (collagen building) and K, Niacin and Potassium; and* **Carrot** *– Vitamins A and K, Coenzyme Q10 and Niacin* **revive skin.**

**Piece of Fruit**
THE SKIN SECRET: *Apple – Vitamins A (skin regenerating) and C (collagen building);* **Banana** *– Potassium, Vitamins A and C.*

# POINTS TO REMEMBER FOR TIGHTER, BRIGHTER, HEALTHIER SKIN

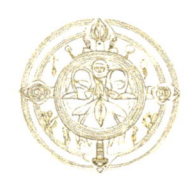

- When it comes to your skin you deserve to give it the best
- Avoid packaged and processed foods as they are full of preservatives, not nutrients
- Alcohol deprives skin of essential vitamins and minerals
- Caffeine is a diuretic and dehydrates the skin
- Smoking dehydrates the skin
- Sugar weakens collagen
- Avoid table salt and use fresh herbs, spices and sea salt instead
- Chew food slowly as good digestion allows nutrients to be absorbed more easily
- Remove excessive saturated fats
- Include raw vegetables in your salad
- If you can't see where or what it comes from, don't eat it

- When our bodies are starved from nutrition we overeat; and while junk food tastes good it is lacking in nutrition
- Eat brown rice instead of white as it is whole and unprocessed
- Never use aluminium pots to cook in
- If you don't eat fish take fish oil supplement capsules
- If you are eating bread, make it whole grain
- Drink plenty of water and eat foods with high water content as it helps cleanse intestines and nourish your body
- Avoid stress as much as possible
- Massage and exercise your face not just your body
- Get eight hours sleep
- Avoid excessive sun exposure
- Give things up gradually rather than force yourself by setting unrealistic goals that you won't keep, as lasting results will be attained with commitment
- Remember your mind is the steering wheel of your life. Whatever you think and believe to be true will become your reality
- Mother nature is the most powerful and effective way to tighten and brighten skin

# FACE LIFTING FOOD LIST

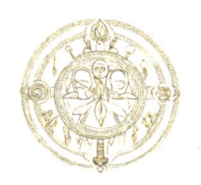

*When we are accepting and happy inside our skin our beauty has depth, meaning and power that multiplies and magnifies our truest selves.*

### FACE LIFTING FRUIT

**Apple** – strong antioxidant properties with Vitamins A, C (collagen building)

**Avocado** - 25 essential nutrients and Vitamins including high levels of Vitamins E and K

**Banana** – antioxidants, Potassium, Vitamins A, B, C

**Berries** – strong antioxidants, high in Vitamins A and C (collagen building) with skin building minerals such as calcium and potassium. The strongest antioxidant of the berry family is blackcurrants which have one of the highest sources of Vitamin C (collagen building)

**Cantaloupe** – extremely high in Vitamins A and C (collagen building)

**Citrus Fruit** – high in Vitamin C (collagen building)

**Currants** – high in Vitamin C and Potassium

**Dates** – high in Vitamin C, Potassium, Phosphorous and Calcium

**Grapes** – high in Vitamin C (collagen building)

**Grapefruit** – extremely high in Vitamins A and C and Potassium

**Guava** – high in Vitamins A and C

**Kiwifruit** – extremely high in Vitamin C (collagen building) and Potassium

**Lemon** – high in Vitamin C (collagen building), Potassium and Calcium

**Mango** – high in Vitamins A, C, E and K

**Nectarine** – high in Vitamins A, C and K

**Orange** – high in Vitamin C (collagen building) with Vitamin A and Potassium

**Papaya** – Potassium, Vitamins A, C (collagen building), E and K

**Passion fruit** – high in Vitamins A and C and Potassium

**Peach** – antioxidant with Vitamins A, E and K

**Pear** – high in Vitamins C and K

**Pineapple** – high in Vitamin C (collagen building)

**Plum** – high in Potassium and Vitamins A, C and K

**Rhubarb** – high in Vitamins C and K and Potassium

**Strawberries** – strong antioxidant high in Vitamins K and C (collagen building) and Potassium

**Tomatoes** – Potassium, Vitamins A and C (collagen building)

**Watermelon** – high in the super antioxidant lycopene and Vitamins A and C (collagen building)

---

## FACE LIFTING VEGETABLES, LEGUMES & OILS

**Alfalfa Sprouts** – high in Vitamins C, K and A, and Zinc

**Artichoke** – high in Vitamins C and K, Potassium, Niacin and Magnesium

**Asparagus** – high in Vitamins A, C and K, Zinc, Potassium, Niacin and Selenium

**Beans** (dried) – Potassium, Zinc and Niacin

**Beets** – Vitamins A and C, Phosphorous, Calcium and Magnesium

**Bok Choy** – extremely high in Vitamins A, C and K, Calcium, Niacin and Potassium

**Broccoli** – high in Vitamins A, C and K and potassium

**Brussels Sprouts** – high in Vitamins A, C and K with potassium

**Butternut Squash** – high in Vitamins A and C with potassium

**Cabbage** – Vitamins A, C and K

**Carrots** – high in Vitamins A and K with Coenzyme Q10 and Niacin

**Cauliflower** – high in Vitamins C and K, Potassium and Niacin

**Celery** – Potassium, Niacin, Vitamins A, C, K

**Cucumber** – strong antioxidant with Vitamins A and C (collagen building) and a number of trace minerals and enzymes

**Eggplant** – high in Potassium, Niacin and Vitamin C

**Garlic** – high in Vitamin C and Selenium

**Ginger** – anti-inflammatory with Zinc

**Green beans** – high in Potassium, Phosphorus and Zinc

**Green and red peppers** – high in Vitamins C (collagen building) and K

**Leek** – high in Vitamins A and K

**Lettuce** – Vitamin C, Beta carotene, Niacin, Potassium

**Lima beans** – high in Zinc, Potassium and Phosphorus

**Mushroom** – Potassium, Vitamins D, B

**Okra** – high in Zinc and Vitamins A, C (collagen building) and K

**Olive Oil** – strong antioxidant and anti-inflammatory high in Vitamins E and K

**Onion** – Vitamin C (collagen building)

**Peas** – high in Vitamins A, C (collagen building) and K, Zinc and Potassium

**Potato** – high in Vitamin C (collagen building), Potassium and Zinc

**Parsnip** – high in Vitamin C (collagen building) and Potassium

**Pumpkin** – high in Vitamins A and C (collagen building) and Potassium

**Radish** – high in Vitamin C (collagen building)

**Spinach** – high in Vitamin A with strong anti-inflammatory antioxidants, Beta Carotene, Vitamins B, C, E and K

**Spirulina** (seaweed) – high in Vitamins A, C and K, Potassium, Magnesium, and Zinc

**Spring onion** – high in Vitamins A, C and K, and Potassium

**Sunflower Oil** – Vitamins A, D, E

**Sweet potato** – high in Vitamin C (collagen building) and Potassium

**Turnip** – high in Vitamin C (collagen building), Niacin and potassium.

**Vegetable Oils** – (Apricot Kernel, Avocado, Almond, Peach Kernel, Jojoba, Sunflower, Sesame, Olive or Soybean) - rich in unsaturated Fatty Acids, Vitamins and minerals

**Yellow squash** – Vitamins A, C, K

**Zucchini** (summer squash) – Vitamins A, C and K, Zinc and Potassium

## FACE LIFTING DAIRY

**Milk** – Vitamins A and D, Niacin and a number of essential skin building minerals

**Yoghurt** – Vitamin A, Niacin, Calcium

**Cheese** – Vitamin A, Calcium

## FACE LIFTING WHOLE GRAINS

**Barley** – Barley is full of antioxidants and enzymes together with Vitamins A, B, C and E

**Oatmeal** – Magnesium, Selenium, Vitamin A

**Rye** – Potassium, Zinc, Selenium

**Whole wheat** – Selenium, Niacin

**Brown Rice** – Niacin, Vitamin B7, Selenium, Magnesium, Potassium, Omega fatty acids

## FACE LIFTING FISH, CHICKEN & MEAT

**Chicken** – Selenium, Vitamin E, Zinc, Proline, Lysine

**Eggs** – Vitamins A, B7, D, Proline, Lysine

**Oily fish** – Omega-3 and 6, Vitamin A, B

**Salmon** – DMAE, Vitamins A, D, Niacin, Calcium, Zinc, Magnesium

**Trout** – Selenium, Magnesium, Niacin, Omega-3, Calcium

**Tuna** – Selenium, Magnesium, Niacin, Omega-3, Potassium

**Lean red meat** – Niacin

---

## FACE LIFTING HERBS & SPICES

**Basil** – Potassium, Beta carotene and Vitamins A and C

**Bay leaves** – Potassium, Vitamins A and C Cumin – Niacin, Potassium and Vitamin A

**Chives** – Potassium, Vitamins A, B and C

**Coriander** – Vitamins A, C, K and Potassium

**Dill** – Potassium, Zinc and Vitamin C

**Lemon grass** – Zinc and Potassium

**Oregano** – Potassium, Zinc, Copper, Niacin, Vitamins A and C

**Parsley** – strong antioxidant properties, high in Vitamins A, C and K

**Rosemary** – Vitamin A, C, E and K, Beta carotene and Niacin

**Tarragon** – Vitamin C and Vitamin A

**Turmeric** – a natural antibiotic, a strong antioxidant and an anti- inflammatory

---

## FACE LIFTING NUTS & SEEDS

**Almonds** – Potassium, Vitamin E

**Flax seeds** – Omega 3, Magnesium, Zinc

**Peanuts** – Vitamin E, Niacin, Copper, Potassium, Zinc

**Pumpkin seeds** – Niacin, Copper, Omega-3

**Sunflower seeds** – Vitamin E, Niacin, Selenium, Copper, Omega-3

**Walnuts** – Zinc, Magnesium, antioxidants , Omega-3

---

## OTHER

**Honey** – antioxidants and low doses of both vitamins and essential minerals

**Tea** – contains antioxidants (antioxidants are neutralised if tea is taken with milk)

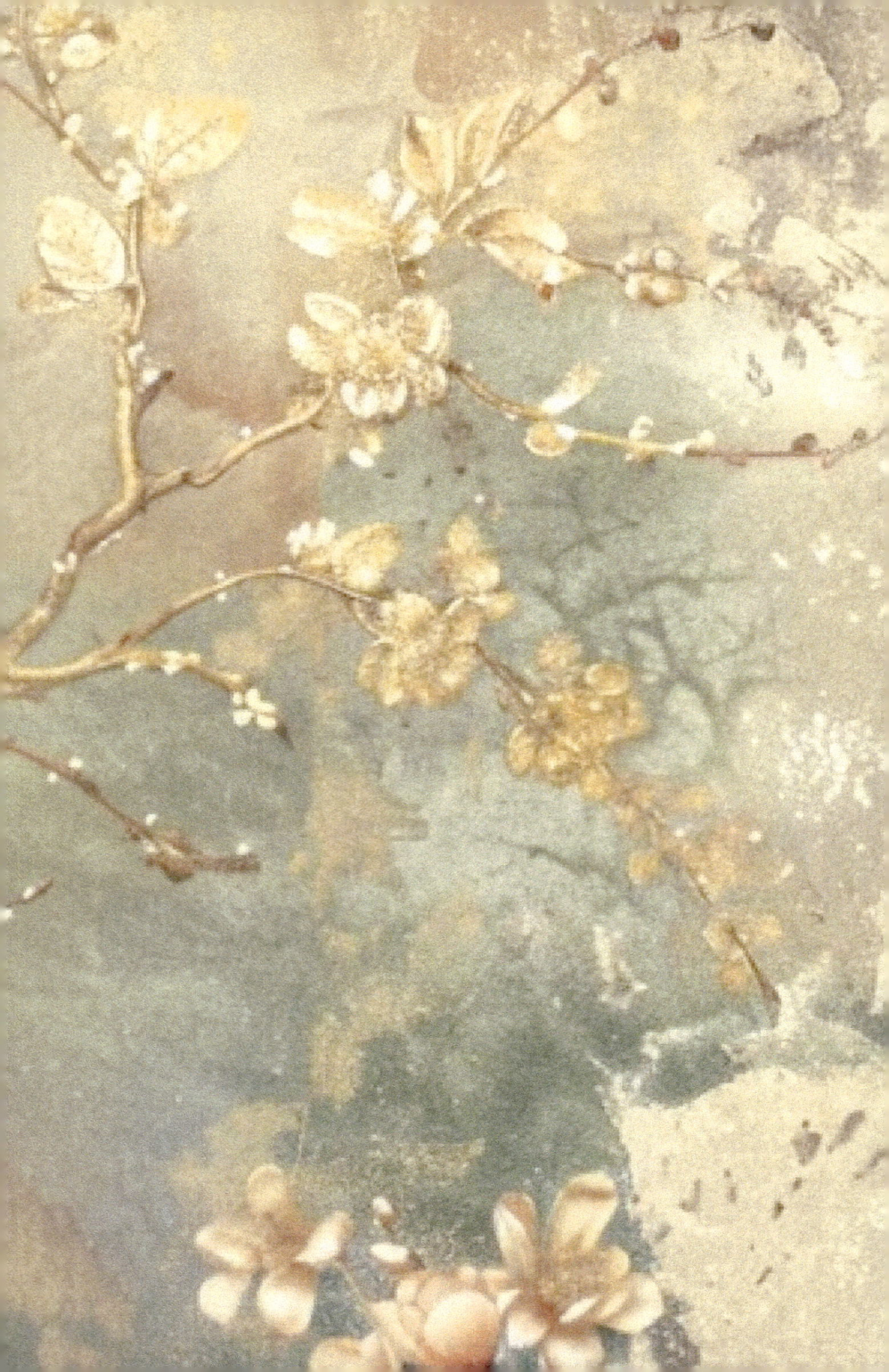

# THE BALANCE OF BEAUTY PHILOSOPHY

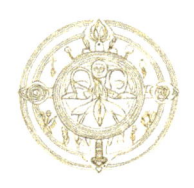

*What we eat has a direct impact not only on how we look, but how we feel.*

*Balance*
*Enthusiasm*
*Acceptance*
*Understanding*
*Trust*
*and You...*

*are the keys to a good life.*

Everyday we are bombarded with a concept of beauty where flawless, 'poreless', wrinkle-free skin is shown as the perfect ideal. The myriad of unrealistic physical standards that have created untold stress, have left people questioning themselves and their beauty - Young enough, pretty enough, thin enough - ENOUGH ALREADY!

These six keys support you to take the stress out of beauty.

They are a testament to the truth of beauty and a celebration of beauty in its truest sense.

BALANCE

**Balance is not about indulgence or repression, but in seeking balance we are encouraged to look closely at the relationship we have with ourselves so that we can begin to live in a balanced way, physically, emotionally, mentally and spiritually.**

- Use your body to live your beauty, your heart to feel it, your eyes to see it, your ears to hear it, your mouth to speak it and your hands to share it.
- Practice wholeness - eat and exercise to increase the flow of energy and nurture wholesome emotions.
- Breathe deeply, it supports your nervous system to relax and helps alleviate anxiety.
- Never settle for less than you know in your heart you really deserve.

## ENTHUSIASM

**Awakening the enthusiastic response within yourself is not about excitement but a deep conviction that what you are and represent is a true reflection of you. The more enthusiasm we feel for ourselves, the more energy we have to participate in life and the more we can express ourselves fully.**

- Put your heart into everything that you do and remain true to yourself.
- Admire others but never envy them.
- Maintain a sense of humour and practice forgiveness.
- Never argue for your limitations only your possibilities.
- Believe in your dreams and don't be afraid to follow them even if no one else will.

## ACCEPTANCE

**Acceptance dissolves the limitations and expectations we have on ourselves and others. Self acceptance is the way we make peace with ourselves. It is not about reciting affirmations or chanting mantras, it is about making the decision to drop judgment from our lives.**

- Keep good company with yourself and practice sitting in silence for at least ten minutes every day.
- Think only beauty when you look into a person's

eyes, and you will begin to see it when you look into your own.
- Make peace with yourself by giving up self criticism and criticism of others.
- Never be scared to say 'no', as you train people how to treat you by what you allow them to do to you.
- Always stand up for your individuality knowing that the key to your happiness is in holding deep convictions about who you are and what you believe.

UNDERSTANDING

**Understanding ourselves gives us emotional and mental clarity, and enables us to honour who we are and the choices we make. Through understanding we begin to open up clear channels of communication with ourselves and others which naturally opens up the way to live authentically.**

- Remember that your beauty is not determined by your bone structure but the structure of your thoughts.
- Concentrate not on how others treat you, but on how you treat yourself.
- Never judge others by their looks, as good looks do not necessarily equate to 'good people' or good love.
- Always choose to be kind – what you give will live in your heart forever.
- Love who you are and all aspects of yourself and don't give that responsibility to anyone else.

TRUST

**Trust attunes our hearts and minds so that we can strengthen self belief and develop spontaneity, creativity and adventure in our lives.**

- Remember that the most beautiful aspect of a human being can't always be seen with your eyes – your heart is one of them.
- Recognise beauty in the things that you do, not only in the things you have.
- Count your blessings and focus on what you have to give the world, rather than what the world has not given you.
- Remember each day that you are whole and beautiful for no other reason than you are human.

YOU

You are the way that love becomes human.
You give it a quality that can be touched and shared.
You give love and life meaning.
Use your body to express this love.
Use your heart to feel it, your eyes to see it, your ears to hear it, your hands to create and share it, and your feet to be grounded in it.
Take a deep breath, kick off your shoes and feel the earth under your feet.
Feel the sun and smell the air.
Fill your eyes with smiling clouds, listen to the birds and

celebrate the body that continually allows you to taste the goodness and richness of life.

**It is time to awaken to the BEAUTY we all possess as human beings, to embrace and experience ourselves in a loving and fulfilling way.**

# THE FOUR PILLARS OF SKIN HEALTH TO DE-STRESS & AGE LESS

## GREGORY LANDSMAN'S PROVEN APPROACH TO ACHIEVE VITAL HEALTHY YOUNGER LOOKING SKIN

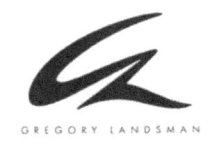

GREGORY LANDSMAN

**If You Are Stressed, So Is Your Skin!**

Stress creates skin stress, which dries the skin and makes you look older than you are. This means that one of the greatest things we can do for our skin is to reduce the stress we experience from day-to-day living.

This four-pronged method helps to stop premature skin aging by purging the body from the internal and lifestyle driven stress that create free radicals and destroys the skin's building blocks, collagen and elastin. Dealing with stress fortifies the body's defence system and supports collagen production, which results in healthier, more vital looking skin at every age. It also increases feelings of wellbeing, which means we look better and feel better.

*I am going to show you how to break the skin stress cycle and stop premature aging and restore skin health, radiance and vitality without any expensive creams, invasive procedures, fillers or botox.*

*While we all want to look as good as we can for as long as we can, we do not have to hurt ourselves to do it. There is no need to wage war on wrinkles, as when we understand how to use the four pillars to skin health to break the skin stress cycle, looking after our skin becomes much easier than we have been led to believe.*

— GREGORY LANDSMAN


## THE FOUR PILLARS OF SKIN HEALTH TO DE-STRESS & AGE LESS

**PILLAR 1: Restore the elasticity and firmness of your skin with facial massage and exercise - see FACE FITNESS: The 10 Minute Face Lift**

**FACE FITNESS** shows you how to exercise and massage the face to lift facial muscles; firm skin; plump up fine lines and regenerate collagen growth; speed up the lymphatic drainage; oxygenate the blood; and remove toxins... an effective way to counteract skin stress and age less naturally.

**PILLAR 2: Elevate your skins radiance and health with food - see FACE FOOD**

**FACE FOOD** shows you how to plump up skin; smooth

out fine lines; boost collagen production; hydrate skin; and get a healthy natural glow from the inside out by eating the right foods. It reveals where to find the powerful anti-aging ingredients such as retinol, alpha hydroxy acid, ferulic acid and hyaluronic acid in the foods we eat. You can eat your way to tighter, brighter, younger looking skin. A powerful way to de-stress skin and age less naturally.

*The science of beautiful skin lies in the foods we eat.*

**PILLAR 3: Transform your skin's glow with active, botanical purity - see FACE VALUE: Save Your Money & Your Skin with Professional, Active, DIY Botanical Skincare.**

The DIY plant powered active formulas in **FACE VALUE** show you that with nature, knowledge and know how, you can take years off your face naturally and feed your skin the purity and goodness it needs to boost skin health, smooth out fine lines, and counteract the impacts of skin stress and the daily use of cosmetics.

It will show you where to find powerful active, botanical skin ingredients used in expensive skin creams and treatments, including retinol, alpha hydroxy acid, ferulic acid and hyaluronic acid from ingredients found in your kitchen. For example, catacalase, is a skin brightening enzyme used in premium priced skincare, that can be found in the juice of the simple potato. **FACE VALUE** delivers an effective way to boost your skin health, reduce skin stress and age less naturally.

*Revive your skin's glow with the gentle touch of nature's active purity and power.*

**PILLAR 4: Unlock the health and vitality of your skin - see STOP THE BIG WRINKLE LIE**

**Discover how to elevate your skin, stop the wrinkle causing hormone & take years off the face naturally with the power of your breath.**

**STOP THE BIG WRINKLE LIE** shows you how changing the way you breathe can change the quality and texture of your skin, restoring skin health and radiance from the inside out. With the power of your breath you can reduce skin stress and age less naturally.

*When you change the way you breathe, eat cortisol lowering foods, use potent active vitamin rich botanical skincare formulas and stimulate the facial muscles, you will revive, renew and repair your skin...at any age.*

*The key to maintaining skin health over a lifetime is to make small changes that counteract skin stress and deliver big skin results when practised regularly.*

*With nature, knowledge and know-how you have the ability to transform the quality and texture of your skin at any age.*

Gregory Landsman

# ABOUT GREGORY LANDSMAN

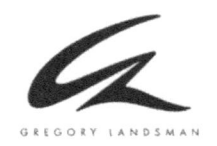

BEST SELLING AUTHOR
GLOBAL BEAUTY & WELLNESS EXPERT
TV HOST

Having spent more than 35 years in the global beauty industry Gregory Landsman is one of the most noted beauty and wellness experts in the world and a best selling author of nine books on how to counteract skin stress and age less.

His science-based and easy to use techniques known as the GL De-Stress & Age Less Method™ are used in universities, recommended by doctors, and shared with global audiences through his books, and TV show *Face Lifting Food*, shown in more than 80 countries worldwide.

Gregory Landsman is also the CEO of the GL Skinfit Institute®.

## CONNECT WITH GREGORY LANDSMAN

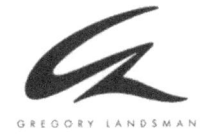

If you would like to hear from me personally with updates, insights, stories and tips on how to reduce skin stress and age less please go to gregorylandsman.com and sign up. I look forward to you joining us.

Gregory Landsman official website:

# NOTES

# NOTES

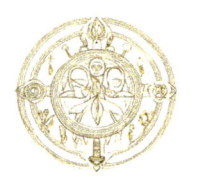

www.ingramcontent.com/pod-product-compliance
Ingram Content Group UK Ltd.
Pitfield, Milton Keynes, MK11 3LW, UK
UKHW050745050525
5760UKWH00043B/453